The Optician
Training Manual

The Optician Training Manual

Simple Steps to Becoming a Great Optician

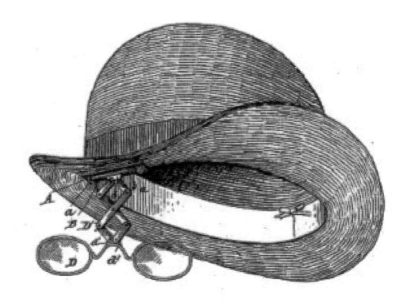

David S. McCleary

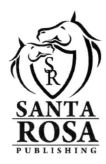

Santa Rosa Publishing,
43980 Mahlon Vail Circle, Suite 206
Temecula, CA 92592. USA

www.santarosapublishing.com

Illustrator: Peter Kyprianou
Book designer: Jonathan Gullery

ISBN number 978-0-578-20676-9

Eyecare is an ever-changing field. Be sure to read product inserts and
dispensing instructions prior to prescribing any product or medication.
Care has been taken to insure proper techniques have been described
within this book, however, it is the responsibility of the prescriber and/or
dispenser to to assess the best possible treatment options for an individual
patient. Neither the publisher nor author assumses any liability for any
injury and/or damage to persons or property arising from the use of this
publication.

At Santa Rosa Publishing we believe every book is indebted to that which
is responsible for its creation. Therefore, a portion of the proceeds of
this book will be contributed to efforts supporting reforestation and
preserving natural resources.

Printed in the United States of America

*To my daughter, Sarah, for her continued inspiration
and patience when Daddy was writing this book
during perfectly good playtime.*

Countless thanks to all my opticians,
past, present, and future,
who helped shape the development of this book.

Contents

CHAPTER HEADINGS PATENT ILLUSTRATION CREDITS

Title Page: Patent 1889; W.H. Brownlow; "Means for attaching eyeglasses to head apparel"

Chapter 1; Patent 1906; Sylvester Slagle; "Eyeglass Lens"

Chapter 2; Patent 1927; E.D. Tillyer; "Ophthalmic lens"

Chapter 3: Patent 1890; Samuel F. Merritt; "Hairpin and holder for eyeglasses"

Chapter 4: Patent 1891; A.B. Lee; "Adjustable sliding clamp for holding glasses"

Chapter 5: Patent 1897; A. Taylor; "Post –visual reflector"

Chapter 6: Patent 1939; Benjamin Welhelm; "Contact lens"

Chapter 7: Patent 1887; Phillip Stevens; "Eyeglass loupe"

Chapter 8: Patent 1903; Andrew Jackson; "Eye-protector for chicken"

Chapter 9: Patent 1879; D.C Ripley ; "Method and Apparatus for forming and finishing ophthalmic glass".

Chapter 10: Patent 1902; George Mansfield; "Pince-nez Eyeglasses"

Introduction

WELCOME! You are beginning your first steps toward becoming an optician, or maybe you are just trying to improve your knowledge about a few key principles. Before you know it, you will be teaching the principles in this book to those who come after you. This book is written for you, the optician who needs to digest clinical relevancy fast in order to hit the floor running and with confidence.

This will be a fun and enjoyable journey through what can be rough waters. As an optician, you will be barraged with patients' wants and needs, putting a strain on your own patience. This book is about navigating through these rough training waters. Its intent is to be your compass. This book is *not* intended to be your sole source of knowledge, however.

This book came about because of the wealth of wonderfully written and detailed texts on opticianry, but the woeful lack of training books to get you, the optician, trained and on the floor quickly and confidently. Your optical manager or team leader is overflowing with knowledge, and you should rely on them heavily for support and help with performing the practice exercises described in this book. Additionally, if your office does not already have a copy, *System for Ophthalmic Dispensing*, by Brooks and Borish, is a wonderful source for supplemental information that falls beyond the scope of this book and should be in every optician's office.

Acquiring the confidence to hit the optical floor running requires the mastery of several key areas. By the time you finish reading this book, these areas should be well ingrained. The primary means of this, however, is by following the exercises in this book. Reading alone is not enough to learn these skills; only through practice will these skills become second nature to you. Perfection is not possible, but through its pursuit we can achieve excellence.

Congratulations on the start, or the continuation, of your journey!

Preface

TRAINING opticians, new and seasoned, is a daunting task. What is the minimum they must know before you let them loose with their first patient? How do you make sure they have understood their training and can apply it to the appropriate situation? Are seasoned opticians remembering the basic principles that can make a good pair of glasses great? These are the questions this book attempts to answer in a simple, fun, and easily implemented fashion.

Presented in this book is a structured program for training new opticians and refreshing the knowledge of seasoned ones. Optometrists, ophthalmologists, optical team leaders, and optical store managers all will find it equally useful. When used as written, it provides a cycle of training and proficiency sessions. Each chapter covers one particular topic, followed by a proficiency test to measure what was learned.

Searching for an optician training program left me to realize there was a definite lack of organized material available. There are plenty of ABO certification programs available, but much of this information is far too overwhelming, expensive, and wrought with theory and calculations for the practicing optician. Practicing opticians need clinical relevancy—and fast. We want our opticians to be trained and on the floor as quickly as possible, and they want to feel comfortable in that role. It is out of this frustrating search for a concise optician training system that led the writing of this manual, which originates from training opticians at my own practice.

Most of us know intuitively that patients judge the competency of their eye doctors based on the decision-making skills of their opticians, so consistent training is of utmost importance. This book will provide you with an easy-to-follow model of training to make both you and your opticians look good.

Ocular Anatomy and Basic Principles

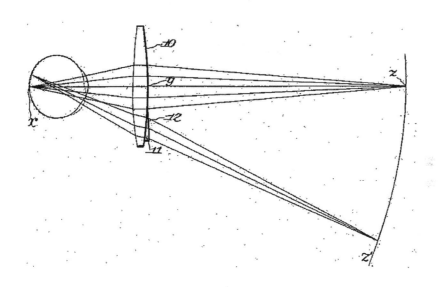

Ocular Anatomy

THE eye is our organ for sight. The anatomy of the eye is composed of an amazingly varied combination of tissues. These tissues do everything from allowing us to process extremely detailed images to warning us of danger before we are even able to identify the threat. And all this in a space of about 23mm. Let us look at the structure and function of this amazing organ.

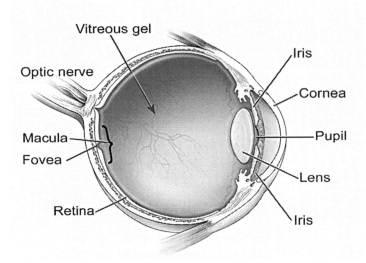

Eye Anatomy (Courtesy: National Eye Institute, National Institutes of Health)

The Cornea: The cornea is the front surface of the eye and has a remarkable trait: it is transparent. This may not seem that amazing, but how many naturally occurring substances can you name that are transparent? In order for the body to create a transparent tissue, it takes an incredibly complex and precise arrangement of fibers made of a substance called *collagen*. Few man-made materials are as transparent as the cornea. The cornea needs to be transparent in order to allow images to pass through to the deeper image-processing layers of the eye.

The Sclera: The sclera is the white of the eye. The sclera provides a tough protective shell and helps the eye maintain its shape.

The Conjunctiva: The conjunctiva is the thin, mostly transparent tissue that overlays the sclera and inner parts of the eyelid. The conjunctiva plays a role in fighting infections (there are a high density of immune-system cells in the conjunctiva), responding to allergens (cells within the conjunctiva are responsible for allergic responses), and maintaining the quality of tears (cells in the conjunctiva produce *mucin*, which helps keep tears in place on the eye.)

The Iris: This is the colored part of the eye. It's similar to the aperture of a camera, and its function is to regulate the amount of light entering the eye. It does this through its control of the *pupil*. The pupil is the opening in the center of the iris through which light enters the eye. Iris muscles pull outward at nighttime or other dark situations to create a larger pupil and therefore allow more light to enter. Similar muscles within the iris constrict to form a smaller pupil in bright light to limit the amount of light entering the eye.

The Lens: The lens is part of the focusing mechanism inside the eye. Tied to your focusing muscles with small string-like fibers called *zonules,* the lens is able to slightly change its shape, and therefore power, in response to how far an object is from the eye. Much like the lens in a camera, this change of focusing power is what enables you to look from a distant object to a near object with ease. Once a person hits the age of forty, however, this lens becomes less flexible, and therefore reading glasses become necessary to do the work that the lens can no longer perform.

The Vitreous: This is the fluid inside the eye. Its role is to create a constant pressure inside the eye that helps maintain the eye's shape and holds the tissues inside the eye in place. The vitreous is composed mostly of water but has a gel-like consistency.

The Retina: Much like film in a camera, the retina is responsible for capturing and processing images. It is the tissue lining the inside of the eye and contains millions of light-sensitive cells called *photoreceptors* (similar to pixels in a digital camera) that respond when stimulated by an image. The central part of the retina, the macula, is used for fine-detail viewing. The peripheral retina, although not as sensitive to details, is well equipped to warn us of oncoming dangers, such as a fast-approaching car from a crossroad.

The Macula: The macula is a term used to describe the part of the retina responsible for fine-detail vision. It is located in the center of the back of the eye and is the part of the retina used when you look directly at an object. The macula contains a much higher concentration of photoreceptor cells than other parts of the retina. This enables you to see much finer details than in other parts of the retina.

The Optic Nerve. The optic nerve is the information superhighway of the eye. It is what collects all the information from the retina, bundles it together, and sends it on to the brain for processing. The optic nerve is what is responsible for everyone's small blind spot, since there are no retinal photoreceptors on the nerve itself.

To find your blind spot, close your left eye and hold your index finger at arm's length in front of your right eye. Look at your fingernail. Now slowly move your arm to your right, keeping your eye fixated straight ahead. After you move your arm about 6–10 inches to your right, you will notice that you no longer see your finger. Keep moving your arm about another inch or two and your finger will suddenly reappear. The same will happen with using your left eye and moving your arm to your left. The point at which your finger disappears is when the image of your finger is falling on the optic nerve entrance into the eye.

Basic Principles

As with any field of study, we must cover a few basics before delving in too deep. These principles will help define some terms and set the stage for principles used later in the book.

What is an image?

An image is nothing more than light reflected from an object, passed through the air, and into our eyes or a camera. If there is no light to shine on an object, does it form an image? No, an image requires a package of light waves reflected from an object.

Just as we cannot hear radio waves unless we have a radio capable of converting the waves into sound, we cannot see images unless we have the right type of reception device. An image is not visible unless two conditions are met:

1. The image is brought to a point of focus (the lens of the eye or a camera is responsible for this); and
2. The image is brought to focus on a surface capable of capturing the

image in a form that is either saved (as on the film of a camera) or instantly processed (as the retina of the eye does).

The light from an object can arrive at the imaging system either from a distant object or from a near object. All objects reflect light in many different directions. If you were to throw a water balloon at an object, the water would bounce from the object in many varying directions; so does light off an object. For a distant object, the imaging system (either the eyeball or a camera) is receiving only light rays that are essentially *parallel* to each other and perpendicular to the imaging device. This is because by the time the non-parallel rays reach the distance of the visual system, they are too far off-course to be captured by the system.

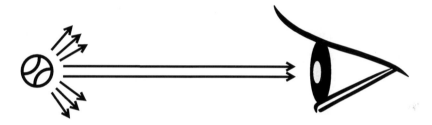

A distant object provides parallel light rays perpendicular
to the imaging system

In comparison, a near object provides *divergent*, non-parallel light rays to the imaging system. This is because the imaging system is close enough to the object to receive these divergent rays. The imaging system is getting wetter from the water balloon because it is closer to the point of impact.

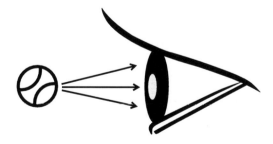

A near object provides divergent light rays to the imaging system

The significance of this difference is in the amount of work the focusing system must do for each type of image. An imaging system requires much more energy to focus divergent rays from a near object than parallel rays from a distant object. This will be discussed in more detail in a following section.

How lenses work

A lens is a transparent material designed to bring an image to a *single point of focus* at a desired distance away from the lens. Why would we want to alter where an image is focused? Because we want to make sure the image falls at the exact location of the image capturing and processing device (such as the film in the case of a camera or the retina in the case of an eye.) Some people have eyes that are a little too short or a little too long for the lens of the eye to overcome, so eyeglass lenses are necessary to make up the difference. By placing the appropriate power lens in front of a person's eye, the lens can do the work that the eye cannot to place the image on the retina.

Lenses bring images to a single point of focus through a process called *refraction*. Refraction occurs whenever images pass through a material of one *index of refraction* and into a material of a different index of refraction. Every material on earth has an index of refraction, including air. Therefore, when an image, or light, is passed from air through a lens, the image will be brought to focus at some distance away from the lens.

Determining exactly how much a lens will refract an image is a measure of the lens's *refracting power*. Increasing the refracting power of a lens means to bring the image to a point of focus closer to the lens itself.

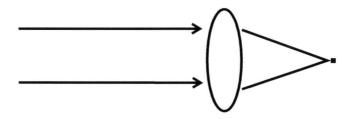

Lens of low refracting power

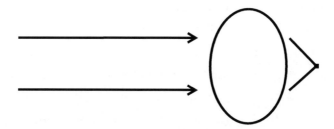

Lens of high refracting power

There are three ways to change the refracting power of a lens:

1. The greater the difference in *indexes of refraction* between the two substances the image passes through, the greater the refracting that occurs. Optically, we think of these two substances as being air and the lens. Air, by the powers that decide these types of things, has been assigned an index value of 1. A lens made from a material with an index of 1.6 is able to refract light better than a lower-index lens, say of 1.4, resulting in a thinner and lighter lens. These types of *high index* lenses will be discussed in a future chapter.
2. The thicker the lens, the greater refracting ability the lens will have if all other factors remain the same.
3. Changing the curvature of a lens can change the refracting ability of the lens, all other things remaining the same.

Let's step back to your childhood for a moment, to reacquaint you with what *point of focus* means. Remember trying to burn a dead leaf with a magnifying glass? Remember how you had to position the magnifying glass at just the right distance from the leaf in order to form a nice tight point of light and therefore maximize your burning potential? What you were doing was finding the point of focus, or *focal point,* of your magnifying lens. The focal point is simply the distance the image is from the lens when the image is perfectly in focus. In this case, you were condensing all of the energy from the sun into a single point. Fortunately, most images we look at do not contain the energy of the sun, and so we are able to see things in focus without spontaneously combusting ourselves. However, looking directly at the sun *will* cause similar damage to the inside of your eye that the magnifier caused to your leaf. Your eye's focusing system, doing just what you are calling upon it to do when you look at the sun, is focusing the energy of the sun into your eye. This will cause a condition known as *solar retinopathy*, a fancy name for saying you burned your eye just like that leaf!

The power of a lens is expressed in units of **diopters.** Just as distances can be measured in miles and temperatures in Fahrenheit, powers of lenses are measured in diopters (often abbreviated simply by a capital D). The higher the diopters of a lens, the stronger the lens's refracting power, and, therefore, the shorter the focal distance of the image from the lens. This relationship is expressed by the equation:

F=1/d

1. *F* is the power of the lens (in *diopters*). If it helps you to remember any easier, simply replace this with a capital *D* for diopters.
2. The *small d* is the distance of the focal point from the lens, measured in meters.

   There are only two simple equations that are important to know from this book, and this is one of them.

For example, a +1.00 diopter lens will focus an image at:

   1=1/d

   Solve for *d* and you get 1 meter. A 1-diopter lens will focus an image 1 meter from the lens.

Now let's look at a higher-power lens, one with a power of +10.00:

   10=1/d

   Solve for d and you get 0.1 meters, or 10 centimeters.

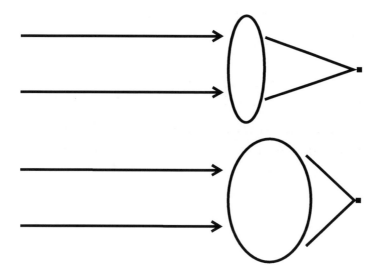

Focal length of +1.00 lens (top) vs. a +10.00 lens (bottom)

So you can see that the higher the power lens, the shorter the focal length.

There are two types of lenses, plus (+) power and minus (-) power. Plus-power lenses bring images to a focus behind the lens. The image formed is called a *real* image. This is the type of lens we are most familiar with, the type that was in your magnifying glass when you tried to burn that leaf. A (+) plus-power lens is a lens that is thicker in the middle than on the edges.

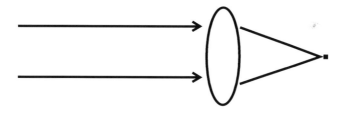

A plus (+) power lens

There is also the (-) power lens, which you will work with often. This lens has a focal point in front of the lens and causes light to disperse instead of come together as it passes through the lens. The image formed is called a *virtual* image. Using our previous equation $F=1/d$, you will notice that if you have a (-) power lens, your answer for the focal distance (d) will be a (-) number as well. What does a (-) answer imply? That the image (called a *virtual image*) will fall in front of the lens instead of behind it. A minus-power lens is thicker on the edges than in the center.

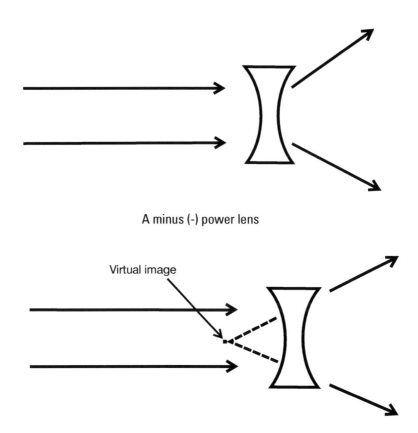

A minus (-) power lens

Virtual image

The virtual image formed by a (-) power lens is found by tracing
the diverging rays backward to their intersection.

The eye has an overall power of about +43 diopters, equivalent to a very strong plus-powered lens. This power helps focus an incoming image at a distance of only 23mm behind the lens onto the retina. Remember the eye is not very long, and so the lens in the eye must be very good at refracting images to have images come into focus so closely behind it.

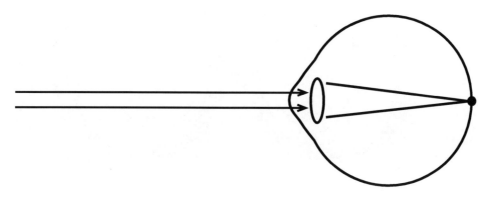

Light rays refracting inside the human eye onto the retina

Types of lenses available

1. Single vision: A single-vision lens is a lens in which the entire lens is set with just one power, or focal point. It is typically used to improve distance vision, but it could be used for reading prescriptions as well.

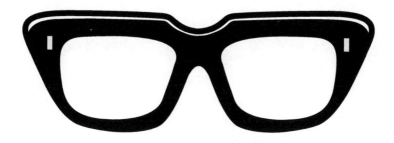

Single-vision pair of glasses

2. Bifocal: A bifocal is a lens with two powers within the same lens. This provides the patient with, for example, a prescription for distance and for reading without needing two different pairs of glasses. This type of lens is typically needed for patients over the age of forty.

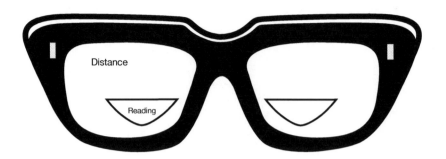

Bifocal

3. Trifocal: A trifocal lens is a lens with three distinct powers: one for distance, one for reading, and one for intermediate tasks. This is typically prescribed for individuals over the age of forty who have a lot of intermediate distance demands throughout their day, such as computer work.

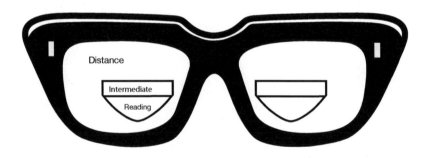

Trifocal

4. Progressive: The progressive lens provides distance, intermediate, and near prescriptions to the patient without the lines inherent in bifocals and trifocals. Progressives incorporate a gradually altering curvature into the lens that slowly adds increasing reading power to patients as they look into the lower parts of the lens. The pitfall? Blending the optics create peripheral distortions in the lens, causing patients not to look through the edge of the lenses but to turn their head to where they want to look. These lenses also are ideal for those patients over the age of forty who have many intermediate-distance visual demands.

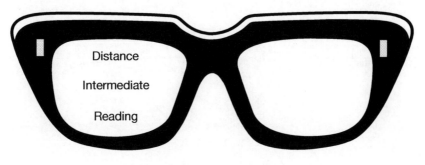

Progressive

How the eye focuses

The eye has an amazingly effective mechanism for bringing images into focus. The lens inside the eye is slightly flexible and is suspended by ligaments called *zonules*. The zonules are in turn connected to the focusing muscles. When an individual is looking at an object in the distance, the muscles are relaxed and the lens is in its "natural" state.

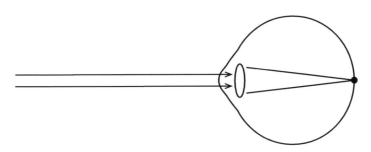

Eye viewing distant object

When an object is brought close to the individual, the image of the object is moved further behind the eye

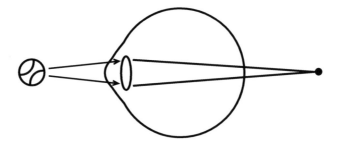

Image falls behind eye with close object

In response to the blur created by not having the image on the retina, the focusing muscles flex, and the lens refocuses on the nearer object. This action is called *accommodation*.

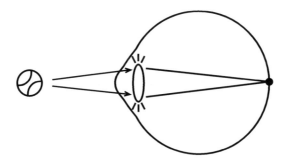

Near object in focus due to flexed muscles

Refractive error

Refractive error is a general term to describe a patient's need for glasses. There are four types of refractive error: myopia, hyperopia, astigmatism, and presbyopia.

1. Myopia: In myopia, or nearsightedness, the images of distant objects fall *in front* of the retina because the eye is too long, creating a blurred image on the retina. A person's lens is unable to correct the focus problem myopia creates. As just discussed, the focusing muscles of the eye can move the image only in one direction—forward—so if the image is already in front of the retina, there is nothing the focusing muscles can do to make it clear.

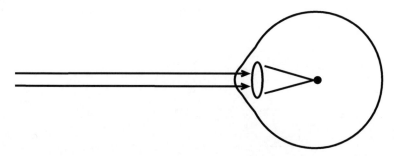

Myopic eye out of focus with distant object

When a myopic person brings an object close to him, the image in the
eye is pushed back to the retina, and the image becomes clear. This is why
we call myopia nearsightedness. A myopic person can see things up close
better than far away.

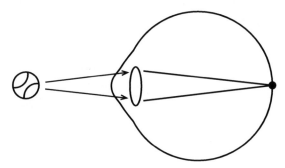

Near object image with Myopia falls on retina

2. Hyperopia: Hyperopia, or farsightedness, is the opposite of myopia.
    In this case, the eyeball is shorter than it needs to be. This creates a
    condition in which the images of distant objects fall behind the retina.

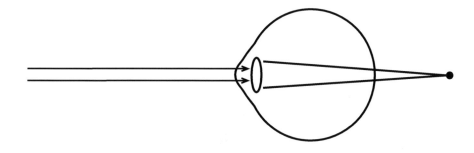

Hyperopic eye

In this case, the focusing muscles in the eye must rise to the occasion and focus to help move the image forward and onto the retina for a clear image.

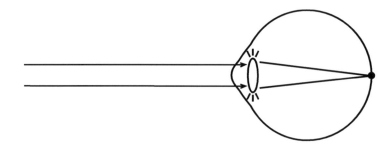

Hyperopic eye bringing distant object into focus

This sounds great, and it is, as long as the person is only slightly farsighted—and young. Just as your muscles get tired when you work out in a gym for a while, your focusing muscles tire as well. This can lead hyperopic patients to develop headaches or blurriness at the end of the day as their focusing muscles give up the fight. The focusing muscles will give up sooner at higher amounts of hyperopia or with increasing age. Over the age of forty, the eye begins to lose its ability to focus, so even those who are slightly farsighted may have blurry vision all day even at distance if they are over forty and are not wearing glasses. Older hyperopes may not get headaches from their farsightedness as younger hyperopes do. Their accommodation muscles are not capable of working hard enough even to create a headache. Older hyperopes will therefore typically complain only of blurriness.

Reading may become difficult for the hyperope as well. Keep in mind that the closer an object gets to the eye, the further behind the eye the image falls, so the more work the focusing muscles must do to bring it forward to the retina. When you are farsighted, the focusing muscles must work hard just to get the image to the retina for distant objects. For near objects, they must work double time.

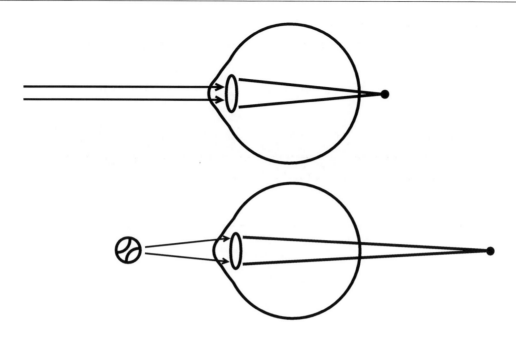

Near object (bottom) creates more work for farsighted
(hyperopic) eye than distant object (top).

3. Astigmatism: Astigmatism is an often-misunderstood word. It is not "a stigmatism," or worse yet, "a stigma," as many patients refer to it. It is "an astigmatism." Astigmatism is simply the state of a cornea that has one axis a little steeper than another axis. This creates a curvature to the cornea resembling a football more than a baseball

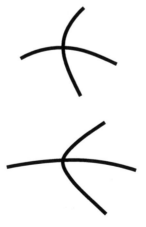

Spherical curvatures (top) and astigmatism curvatures (bottom)

Astigmatism is not a disease or anything bad. In fact, *everyone* has astigmatism to some degree. Just as nothing in nature is perfectly symmetrical, the front of the cornea is not perfectly symmetrical in the vertical and horizontal axis.

Astigmatism is easily corrected with glasses or contact lenses. Without correction, astigmatism may lead to an appearance of double vision, or what is commonly referred to as ghosting.

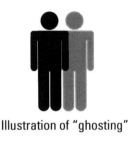

Illustration of "ghosting"

This is the result of the two different corneal curvatures effectively creating two different powers within the eye, or two different images within the eye at slightly different locations.

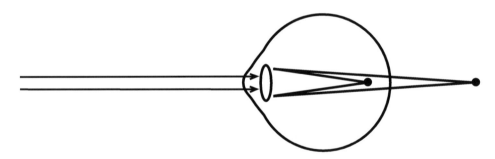

Two focal points in astigmatism

4. Presbyopia: *Hey, my arms aren't long enough anymore!* This is the battle cry of people over forty. Presbyopia is the reason, and it is the condition that strikes everyone without prejudice around the age of forty. The exact mechanism is still being debated, but essentially the eye loses its ability to focus on near objects. The loss of ability is subtle at first, but progresses over the course of the next thirty years to a point at which patients have no ability to focus on near objects without the help of corrective glasses.

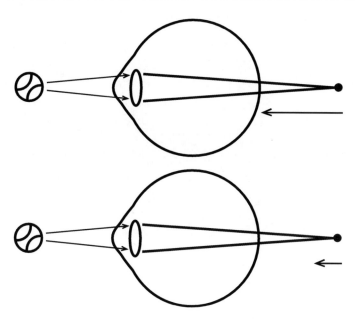

Pre-presbyopia (top) and presbyopia (bottom) focusing ability on near objects

There are two competing theories as to why this happens. One is that the focusing muscles lose their strength and therefore are less able to change the shape of the lens. The second theory is that the lens hardens with time, and by age forty, it is hardened enough to reduce its ability to change shape to bring near objects to focus. The answer probably lies a little with both theories.

Once presbyopia strikes, there are a few possible outcomes.

1. If the patient is emmetropic (does not need distance glasses): This patient will just wear a pair of plus-power reading glasses for near tasks. (Recall that a plus-power lens will shorten the focal point, bringing the near object to the retina.)

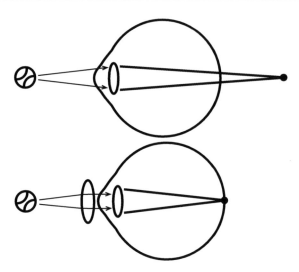

Effect of presbyopia without (top) and with (bottom)
a plus-power reading glass

2. If the patient is myopic or hyperopic, requiring a distance
    correction: This patient will likely decide on a bifocal. As you
    recall, this lens has two powers, one on top for distance tasks and
    one on the bottom for near tasks. A bifocal is often chosen for
    convenience so that these patients will not need to carry two pairs
    of glasses, a distance and a near pair, with them all the time.

3. If the patient is myopic: These patients may choose simply to take
    their distance glasses off to read, as their eyes are naturally focused
    for near tasks without any correction. They may also choose a
    bifocal so they do not need to constantly take their glasses on and
    off throughout the day. Myopes will often say, "But I can read just
    fine without glasses; why do I need a bifocal?" They do not—as
    long as they are willing to take their glasses off every time they
    want to read. Distance glasses alone will not allow the forty-plus-
    year-old myope to read. To the contrary, distance glasses alone
    will neutralize the myope's natural nearsightedness and impede
    reading ability as long as the glasses are bring worn.

Summary of Refractive Errors and Their Symptoms

REFRACTIVE ERROR	SYMPTOM
Myopia	Blurry distance vision
Hyperopia	Blur and headaches when reading (if under age 40) Blur in distance and with reading (if over age 40)
Astigmatism	Blur in distance and with reading. Possible ghosting of images if astigmatism is severe enough.
Presbyopia	Patient over forty with a complaint of decreased reading vision.

How lenses are used to correct refractive error:

When we refer to an eye being too short or too long, and therefore needing corrective glasses to make up the difference, we are talking about microscopic measurements. An eye needs to be only 1mm too long in order to be moderately nearsighted. Using the knowledge we now have about how plus- and minus-power lenses move an image, we can see what power lens a myopic or hyperopic person would need to correct their vision. It is best to think in terms of whether we want to add overall (+) plus-power to the system and therefore shorten the focal distance or take away overall (+) power and move the focal point further away.

In myopia, since the eyeball is longer than it needs to be, we need a lens that would extend the image distance. A (-) minus-power lens would reduce the overall plus power of the eye and therefore lengthen the distance at which the image is focused.

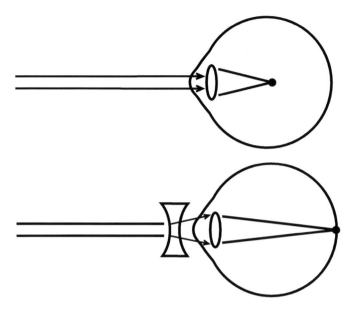

Minus-power lens moving image to the retina in myopia

What power lens would be required to correct hyperopia? If the image is falling behind the retina and we want to move the image to the retina, we need to add *more* plus (+) power to the system, and a (+) plus-power lens would do this for us.

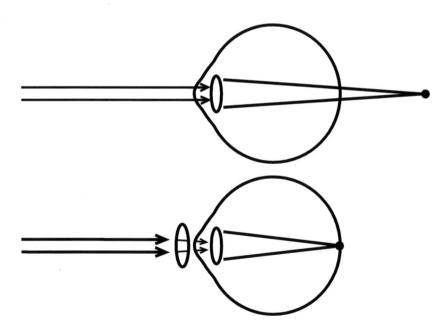

Plus lens moving an image to the retina in hyperopia

Again, keep in mind that plus and minus corrective eyeglass lenses are making a small adjustment to the eyes' natural plus-powered system. A minus power eyeglass lens reduces the overall plus and pushes the image toward the retina. A plus-power lens adds a slight amount of additional plus power to the eye and brings the image back to the retina of a short eye.

Bifocals help compensate for a person's loss of focusing ability after the age of forty. At any age, a person needs an additional 2.5 diopters of plus power to focus on near objects compared to distance objects. Under age forty, there is more than enough strength, or *accommodation* ability, in the focusing system to do this. After age forty, this begins to decline in a very predictable fashion.

Let us look at a pre-forty-year-old's ability to focus on a near object.

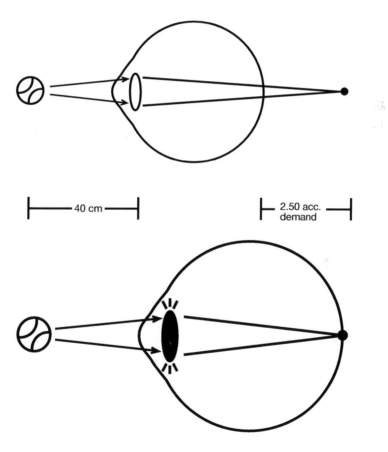

A pre-forty-year-old focusing system overcoming an accommodation demand to focus on an object

The focusing muscles in the eye of a pre-forty-year-old are more than capable of meeting the near focusing demand.

Let's now look at a forty-five-year-old's focusing system

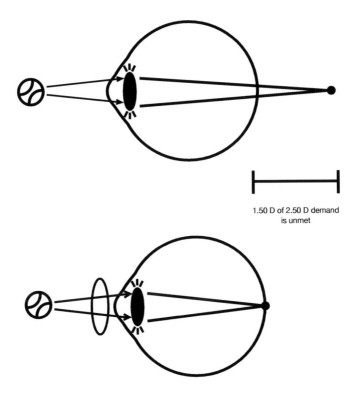

1.50 D of 2.50 D demand
is unmet

A 45-year-old focusing system can do only 1.0D of 2.5D of required work.
Reading glasses are necessary to finish the job.

Here, the patient's focusing system is able to support only about half of the demand, or 1.50 diopters. Therefore, this patient would need a 1.00 diopter add to make up the difference.

Let us now look at a seventy-year-old's focusing system:

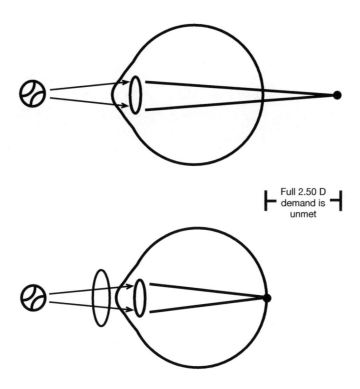

A seventy-year-old cannot meet any of 2.5D demand. Reading glasses or bifocal of power +2.50 is necessary to focus on a near object.

Seventy-year-olds have no power left in their focusing systems. Their bifocals must be a +2.50 to do all of the work that the seventy-year-old focusing system is no longer able to do.

In reality, people never lose *all* of their focusing ability, but the human focusing system is not capable of working at 100 percent, either. Although these examples are slightly simplistic, they should help you understand the need for bifocals in individuals over forty

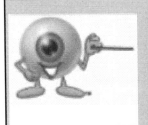 **Focus point:** Glasses do not magnify. You will often have patients ask if their glasses can be made stronger so they can see better. The answer is no. Glasses that are too strong will make things just as blurry as glasses that are too weak. The prescription in glasses is intended only to place the clearest image possible on the retina, not to make that image bigger. A condition may exist, such as cataracts, that will keep a particular patient from obtaining as clear an image as someone else has. To make images bigger, you need a magnifier. Magnifiers are available both for distance and near work. Speak with your doctor or team leader if patients are in need of more help than their glasses can provide.

How prescriptions are written

Reading a prescription for the first time can be like reading a foreign language, and that doesn't even factor in a doctor's illegible handwriting. We will now review eyeglass prescriptions so you will be fluent in its language when you see one for the first time.

A prescription has up to four parts:

1) Sphere power
2) Cylinder power (if necessary)
3) Axis of cylinder (if necessary)
4) Add power (if necessary)

This is what a common prescription form may look like:

INLAND EYE SPECIALISTS

HEMET OFFICE
361 N. San Jacinto Street
Hemet, California 92543-3118
Telephone (951) 652-4343

MURRIETA OFFICE
25395 Hancock Avenue, Suite 100
Murrieta, California 92562
Telephone (951) 696-5388

TEMECULA OFFICE
31950 Hwy. 79 So., Suite B7
Temecula, California 92592
Telephone (951) 303-0575

Axis
Cylinder
Sphere
Right Eye
Left Eye
Bifocal Power
Dr's Recommendations

PATIENT _____ DATE _____

℞	Sphere	Cylinder	Axis	Vis. Acuity	VTX	Prism	Base
O.D.				20/			
O.S.				20/			
Add	+						

❏ Bifocal ❏ Trifocal ❏ SV Dist ❏ SV Reading

❏ Sunglasses
❏ AR Coat
❏ Plastic
❏ Polycarbonate
❏ P.A.L.

❏ Probably will not improve vision
❏ UV-400
❏ Photochromatic
❏ Tint of Choice

Remarks:_____

_____

Dr._____

And this is what it looks like completed by a doctor:

INLAND EYE CLINIC MEDICAL GROUP

HEMET OFFICE
361 N. San Jacinto Street
Hemet, California 92543-3118
Telephone (951) 652-4343

MURRIETA OFFICE
25395 Hancock Avenue, Suite 100
Murrieta, California 92562
Telephone (951) 696-5388

TEMECULA OFFICE
31950 Hwy. 79 So., Suite B7
Temecula, California 92592
Telephone (951) 303-0575

PATIENT John Smith DATE 2/15/08

℞	Sphere	Cylinder	Axis	Vis. Acuity	VTX	Prism	Base
O.D.	-1.00	-0.75	180	20/20			
O.S.	-1.50	-1.00	170	20/20			
Add	+2.00						

☑ Bifocal ❏ Trifocal ❏ SV Dist ❏ SV Reading

❏ Sunglasses
(☑ AR Coat)
❏ Plastic
(☑ Polycarbonate)
❏ P.A.L.

❏ Probably will not improve vision
❏ UV-400
❏ Photochromatic
❏ Tint of Choice

Remarks:_____

_____

Dr._____

Let us now look at each entry in detail: Each eye will have its own set of data. *"OD" is the abbreviation for the right eye and "OS" is the abbreviation for the left eye.*

1. Sphere power:

    The sphere power is the amount of myopia or hyperopia. Myopia, as you recall, is corrected with a minus-power lens. Therefore, it will be signified with a (-) sign in front of its sphere power. Hyperopia, because it is corrected by a plus-power lens, will have a (+) sign in front of its power.

2. Cylinder power:

    The cylinder is the amount of astigmatism corrected for in the lens. This can be written in either + or − form. We will discuss shortly how to convert between the two forms. A cylinder creates two different powers within the same lens, just as an astigmatism creates two different powers within the same eye.

    In the rare event that a patient needs no astigmatism correction, this box will simply contain the letters "DS," which stands for *Diopter Sphere,* meaning no cylinder component is needed in the glasses. "Sphere" or "Sph" are other comments that may be written in this box and represent the same as "DS."

3. Axis:

    The axis is the orientation of the cylinder power. You will recall that in astigmatism, the cornea has a steeper and flatter axis. The axis corresponds to the orientation of the flattest or steepest (depending on whether it is written in plus or minus cylinder form) axis of the cornea. Having the correct axis for a person's astigmatism is similar to having the correct orientation of a key to unlock a door. This section would be blank if there is no cylinder component.

4. Add power:

    The add power signifies the power of the bifocal. This is fairly standard for a given age, since nearly all people lose their focusing ability at about the same rate beginning around age forty. For example, nearly all forty-four-year olds will need a +1.25 add, and nearly every seventy-year-old will require a +2.50 add.

The cylinder component of a prescription may be written in either minus or plus power depending on the type of equipment the doctor uses. Typically, optometrists will use minus cylinder instruments, and ophthalmologists will use plus cylinder. Both methods of writing the prescription give you the same result in the glasses; they are just different ways of looking at the same numbers. Depending on where you work, you will probably see the same type of prescription notation every time. However, you will need to know how to convert between the two types of prescription formats in case a patient comes to you from another doctor's office that used the other notation.

To convert from plus to minus cylinder, or vice versa:

1. Add the cylinder to the sphere. This is your new sphere component.
2. Change the sign of the cylinder.
3. Keep the cylinder power the same.
4. Add or subtract 90 degrees to the axis to keep the axis between 1 and 180. To do this, if you start at an axis greater than 90, subtract 90. If you start from an axis less than 90, add 90. There is no such thing as an axis greater than 180; if your math reveals otherwise, recheck your math.

Let us look at a couple of examples:

1. You have a prescription of -1.00 – 1.00 × 180. What is the prescription in plus-cylinder form?
    1. Add cylinder to the sphere (-1.00 + -1.00 = -2.00). This is your new sphere.
    2. Change the sign of the cylinder. The new cylinder is (+).
    3. Keep the cylinder power the same. The cylinder power is still 1.00.
    4. Since we cannot go over 180 degrees, we cannot add 90 to 180; therefore, we will subtract 90 from axis 180 and arrive at axis 90.

Therefore, our translated power is **-2.00 + 1.00 × 090**.

2. You now have a prescription of -2.00 + 2.00 × 040. Convert this into minus cylinder form.

    1. Add the cylinder to the sphere (-2.00 + 2.00 = 0.00) This is your new sphere.

    2. Change the sign of the cylinder. The new cylinder is (-).

    3. Keep the cylinder power the same. The cylinder power is still 2.00.

    4. Since we cannot go below 000 degrees, we cannot subtract 90 from 40; therefore, we will add 90 to axis 40 and arrive at axis 130.

Therefore, our translated power is **0.00 – 2.00 × 130**.

A lens with a power of 0.00D may also be written as "Plano." Therefore, you may see the prior prescription written also as **Plano – 2.00 × 130.**

How vision is measured

Patients will often ask, "So what is my vision?" They are likely referring to the numeric notation given to their visual acuity. Everyone seems to know that 20/20 vision is good, but not many patients know what 20/20 means or if 20/40 is better or worse than 20/20.

When referring to visual acuity in numeric notation, the first number refers to the testing distance. Most visual acuity charts are designed to be used with the patient 20 feet away. The vast majority of visual acuity measurements will have a "20" as the first number to indicate this 20-foot testing distance.

The second number refers to the smallest size letter the patient is able to read at the 20-foot distance. A 20-size letter creates an angle of 5 *minutes of arc* at 20 feet. *Minutes of arc* is simply an angular measurement of the size of the letter. A 40-size letter subtends 10 minutes of arc, a 60-size letter subtends 15 minutes of arc, and so forth. The science behind this angular measurement is beyond the scope of this book, but the important take-home point is that looking at the second number of the acuity notation can tell you how far from 20/20 (perfect) vision the patient has. The larger the second number, the larger the letter needs to be in order for the patient to be able to read it. The size of the letters is scaled proportionally, meaning that a 40-size letter is twice the size of a 20-size letter, a 100-size letter is five times the size of a 20-size letter, and so forth.

Occasionally, in a patient with an ocular disease such as macular degeneration, the patient is not able to see even the largest letter (usually a letter *E*) at 20 feet, so the visual acuity measurements are done at a closer distance. If the big *E* (the

400-size letter), for example, must be moved to 10 feet in front of the patient in order to be read, the visual acuity is recorded as 10/400. This is the equivalent to 20/800, but typically, there is not an 800-size letter on the chart, so the doctor must move the 400-size letter twice as close to give the same effect.

With this knowledge, we can now reason that a person with a visual acuity of 20/80 will need to be four times closer to an object than someone with an acuity of 20/20 in order to see it as well.

You now know the basics of ocular anatomy and optics (assuming you can answer the questions on the next page!) The next chapter will throw you feet-first into what you will be doing for much of your day: analyzing a pair of glasses to determine their accuracy.

Chapter 1 Post Test

1. What is the purpose of the cornea?

2. What is the purpose of the optic nerve?

3. What are the two conditions that must be met in order for an image to be seen?

4. What is the focal length of a lens with a power of +4.00?

5. Name two types of lenses that have three separate powers: one for distance vision, one for intermediate vision, and one for near vision.

6. What is the name of the structure in the eye that is capable of flexing in order to bring images into focus?

7. Ghosting is a common symptom of what refractive error?

8. If a person complains of blurriness when looking at the television but sees well when reading, the most likely diagnosis would be what?

9. What power lens (+ or -) does someone who is hyperopic require?

10. Convert the prescription -4.00 + 1.00 × 090 into MINUS cylinder form.

11. A visual acuity of 20/100 is how much worse than 20/20?

12. Do glasses ever magnify?

CHAPTER 2

Lens Parameters

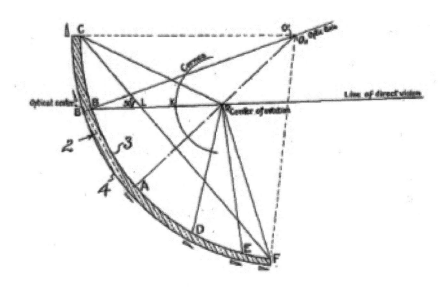

LENS parameters include all aspects of a prescription lens that make it a final product suitable for wearing by the patient. This includes more than just the power of the lens. It also includes the curves, the location of the power, and any aberrations. This chapter is the equivalent of an anatomy class to a future doctor. Here you will learn about and see the inside workings of a lens that your patients will see just as a piece of plastic.

To measure most of the parameters of a lens, you will need an instrument called a *lensometer.* A lensometer will be the instrument you use most often as an optician. The lensometer is used to determine: 1) the sphere power; 2) the cylinder power; 3) the bifocal add power; 4) the axis of the cylinder; 5) the location of the optical center; 6) the amount of prism; and 7) the base direction of the prism.

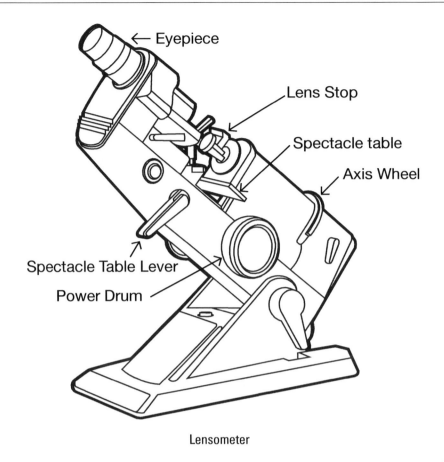

Lensometer

The following is a list of the most commonly used parts of the lensometer. Some of the words may seem unfamiliar now, but we will describe how each is used:

1. Eyepiece: Used to focus the lensometer for the user
2. Lens holder lever: Used to hold eyeglass lenses in place on the instrument through spring-action force
3. Ink marker: Used to dot the optical center location of the lens once it is centered in the lensometer
4. Inkwell: Used to apply ink to the ink marker
5. Spectacle table lever: Used to raise or lower eyeglasses
6. Spectacle table: A resting table for eyeglasses to sit on during measurement
7. Power drum: A measurement dial from which the eyeglass power will be read

8. Lens stop: Tube against which the eyeglass lens is placed in the instrument

9. Cylinder axis wheel: Used to find the axis of cylinder power

Power Measurements

Finding the sphere, cylinder and axis

The power of a lens is the most basic lens parameter—the part that gives the patient the ability to see well. The other parameters we will learn only contribute to this goal. The lensometer will be essential in measuring the power of a pair of glasses.

Depending on where you work, you may become more accustomed to working in either plus-cylinder or minus-cylinder format. We will outline how to use the lensometer in minus cylinder format. In essence, the lensometer simply measures the power in each axis of the lens, so converting from plus- to minus-cylinder will be straightforward.

The steps to measuring the distance power are:

1. Set the *power drum* to 0.00 and look through the *eyepiece*. You will see a circular grid with two sets of perpendicular lines. These lines are called the *mires*. One of the mires is a set of three lines narrowly spaced, the other is a set of three lines more widely spaced, as seen below. Rotate the eyepiece until the mires are clear and in focus.

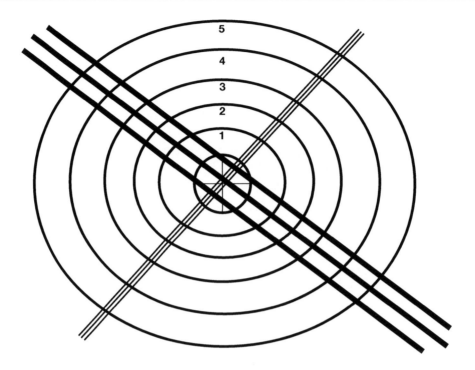

2. Pull the *lens holder lever* fully toward you until it locks into place away
    from the *lens stop.* Place the eyeglasses into the lensometer so that the
    back surface of the lens to be measured is against the lens stop, and the
    eyeglass temples are pointing away from you.

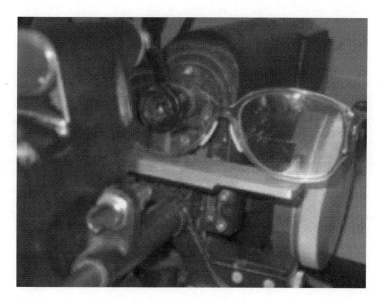

Eyeglasses in lensometer

3. Turn the *power drum* to a power of +10 (black numbers on drum). This
   will give us a starting point likely well outside the actual power of the
   eyeglasses. While looking through the eyepiece, slowly rotate the drum
   toward you (to less plus power) until the mires just begin to come into
   focus.

4. Adjust the spectacle table height so that the center of the mires is in the
   center of the reticle.

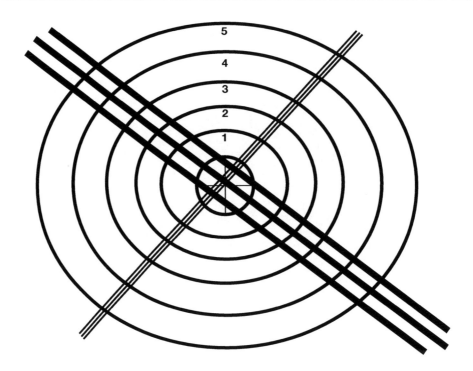

5. Rotate the *cylinder axis wheel.* You will see the mires rotate. Do this until
    the narrow mires becomes a straight line. Continue rotating the power
    drum toward you. When the narrow mire line is both straight *and* clear,
    read the power from the power drum. **This is the sphere power of the
    lens**. If the wide mires come into focus first, you know you are 90 degrees
    off on your cylinder axis wheel. Spin the axis wheel until the narrow
    mires come into focus before the wide mires do.

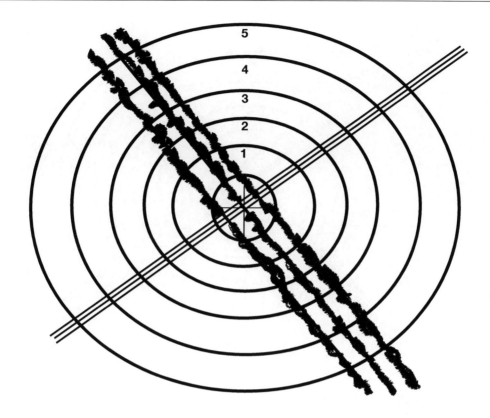

If both the narrow and wide mires come into focus at the same time, and rotating the cylinder axis wheel makes no difference on the apparent straightness of the mires, then you have a spherical lens power, which has no cylinder component.

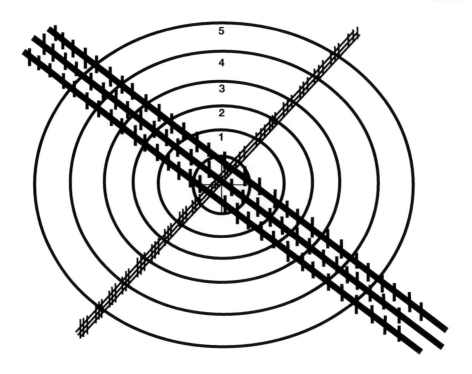

Illustration of mire lines not being straight. An adjustment of the axis is needed.

6. Look back into the eyepiece and continue turning the drum toward you
   until the wide mires comes into focus. You should not need to make any
   adjustments to the cylinder axis wheel. When the wide mires are in focus
   (the narrow mires will now be out of focus), read the corresponding
   power from the power drum. This will be the power 90 degrees away from
   your sphere power. **The cylinder power of the lens is the difference in
   power between when the narrow mires and wide mires were in focus**.

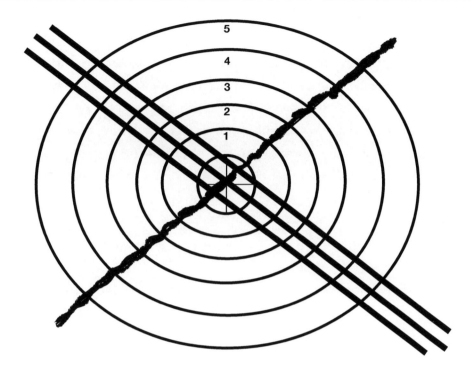

Wide mires now in focus and narrow mires out of focus.

7. Read the axis (in degrees) from the cylinder axis wheel. **This is the axis of the cylinder.**

8. Repeat with the other lens.

You will notice that by starting at a high plus power on the power drum, moving it toward you until the narrow mires are in focus for the sphere power, then moving it toward you again to get the wide mires in focus for the second power, that the second power will be *more minus* then the first power number. Since the cylinder is the difference between the two powers, this method will give you the power in minus cylinder format.

By reversing the rotation of the power drum (starting from a high minus-power and rotating the drum away from you), you will end up with your wide mires in focus at a power *more plus* than your first narrow mires were. Because the cylinder is the difference between the two powers, your cylinder power will be in plus-cylinder format.

Let's look at an example.

After focusing your eyepiece and situating your eyeglasses into the lensometer, you begin your power measurement. You want to measure the power in minus-power format, so you start at +10 on the power drum.

You get your narrow mires straight and in focus at a drum power of +4.00. You continue rotating the drum toward you and find that the wide mires come into focus at a power of +2.00. The axis on your cylinder axis wheel reads 090. What is the power of this lens?

1. The power reading when the narrow mires were straight and in focus is your sphere power: **+4.00.**
2. The difference between the narrow mire power (+4.00) and the wide mire power reading (+2.00) is the amount of cylinder power, **-2.00.**
3. The axis is the number read off the cylinder axis wheel, in this case **090.**

The power of this lens is therefore +4.00 – 2.00 × 090.

Let's look at another example:

After focusing your eyepiece and situating your eyeglasses into the lensometer, you begin your power measurement. You want to measure the power in plus-cylinder format this time, so you start at -10 on the power drum.

You get your narrow mires straight and in focus at a drum power of +1.00. You continue rotating the drum and find that the wide mires come into focus at a power of +2.00. The axis on your cylinder axis wheel reads 130. What is the power of this lens?

4. The power reading when the narrow mires were straight and in focus is your sphere power: **+1.00.**
5. The difference between the narrow mire power (+1.00) and the wide mire power reading (+2.00) is the amount of cylinder power, **+1.00.**
6. The axis is the number read off the cylinder axis wheel, in this case **130.**

The power of this lens is therefore +1.00 + 1.00 × 130.

Finding the bifocal add power

For bifocal lenses, you will also want to know the power of the bifocal. The bifocal will always be more plus in power than the distance part of the prescription. It is called a bifocal "add," as the presence of the bifocal will always *add* more plus power to the prescription to help the patient read.

To find the bifocal add power:

1. As before, place the distance portion of the lens in the lensometer. Rotate the power drum until the most vertical mire is in focus. It does not matter whether this is the narrow or wide mires. Note the power from the power drum.
2. Raise the spectacle table so that the bifocal portion of the lens is now against the lens stop.
3. Look through the eyepiece. The most vertical mire will now be out of focus since a new lens power is now against the lens stop. Rotate the drum until the most vertical mire is in focus again.
4. **The difference in power of the most vertical mire in these two measurements is the amount of the bifocal add.** The bifocal power will always be a (+) power and will usually be a value of between +1.00 and +3.00. The older the individual, the greater the add power you should expect.

To check yourself, the following guidelines should serve as a reminder of approximately what a person's bifocal add power will be, assuming it was prescribed for a standard 16 inch reading distance. If the add power is found to be weaker than expected, the glasses were probably prescribed to be used for some task performed further away than typical reading, such as computer work. Recall from chapter one that a *lower* power lens will have a *longer* focal distance.

Age	Bifocal Add
40-45	+0.75 to +1.50
46-50	+1.50 to +2.00
51-65	+2.00 to +2.25
> 66	+2.50 to +3.00

Here's an example:

> Measuring the power of the most vertical mire in the distance portion of a pair of glasses, you find the power drum to be at a reading of -2.00.
>
> You now slide the spectacle table upward so that the bifocal is against the lens stop. You measure the power of the most vertical mire again and obtain a measurement of 0.00.
>
> What is the power of the bifocal add?
>
> The difference between the two readings, written in plus power, is the bifocal add. Therefore, **the bifocal add in this case is +2.00.**

You will have numerous patients who do not need distance correction and need only a reading prescription. They will often ask you what power-readers they should get from the store. The answer depends on the working distance at which the patient likes to read. Recall that reading glasses do not magnify. All readers can do is provide a clear image at the distance they are prescribed for. The higher the power, the shorter the focal distance of the lens, and therefore the closer the patient will need to hold things to make them clear. The lower the power, the further away the patient can hold things. Both have a benefit. For example, a high-power reading lens may be necessary for reading small print on a medicine bottle, because it allows patients to hold the bottle very close. On the other hand, a weaker power is necessary when the same patients use a computer so they do not need to put their nose up to the monitor.

So why does a high-power reading prescription give the appearance of magnification? The answer is *relative distance magnification.* By allowing the patient to hold material closer to the eyes, it projects a larger image of the object into the eye. This is similar to looking at a person standing across the street and then again seeing the same person standing directly in front of you. Is the person standing in front of you actually more magnified than he was when he was across the street? Of course not, but when he is closer to you, he is creating a larger retinal image size. This gives the appearance of magnification and provides a better appreciation for his details. This differs from a magnifier, because magnifiers do not usually require the person to get closer to the object being viewed.

Seg Height, Seg Width, and Distance Between Segs

Besides the bifocal power, you should be aware of a few other bifocal parameters. These are the seg height, seg width, and distance between segs (DBS). The *seg* is the name of the top edge of the bifocal. These three parameters measure the position of the bifocal in the frame. Ideally, the position is set to maximize its ease of use for the wearer.

Measuring the seg height

The seg height is the distance the bifocal line (the seg) sits above the lowest portion of the lower rim of the glasses. This is measured from the top edge of the lower rim to the bifocal line. To this measurement, add 0.5mm to account for the distance the lens is sitting inside the frame groove. Let's look at an example:

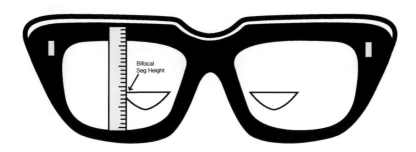

Let's suppose that in this example, the measuring rule lines up with the bifocal seg line at 19mm. Therefore, we would record the seg height as being 19.5mm.

Measuring the seg width

Now let's look at the seg width measurement. Bifocals come in four widths: 28mm, 35mm, 45mm, or executive (all the way across the entire length of the lens). About 95 percent of all the bifocals you see will be the 28mm variety. Unless you specify on your orders, the lab will typically automatically make it this width without calling you to verify. In order to measure the seg width, simply use your measuring rule to measure the bifocal from one edge of the seg line to the opposite edge of the seg line. For example:

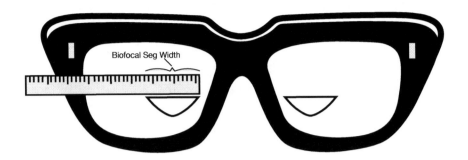

If we set the "0" mark of the ruler on the inner edge of the bifocal seg line, we then read the measurement at the opposite edge. This will be either 28mm, 35mm, or 45mm. If the bifocal line extends all the way across, there is no need to measure; you can assume it is an executive bifocal.

Although the 28mm seg width is the most common, do not hesitate to order a wider seg width for people who spend much of their day reading. Architects or other professionals who need to look at large, spread-out drawings all day especially tend to appreciate some of the wider width bifocals that give them a wider field of view when reading.

Measuring the distance between segs (DBS)

The distance between segs (DBS) of a bifocal is measured as the distance between corresponding parts of the bifocals. Pick a corner of the bifocal, either the left or right, of each lens, and measure the distance between these points.

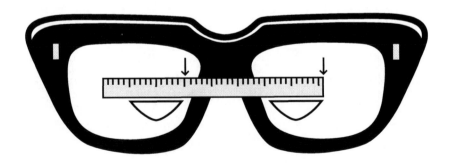

Arrows indicate measurement of Distance Between Segs (DBS)

In this example, if we set the "0" mark of the ruler at the right edge of the bifocal on the left lens, we will read the measurement that lines up with the right edge of the right lens bifocal.

The Optical Center of a Lens

The optical center of a lens is important; it can be thought of as the "sweet spot" of a lens. It is where the optics are the most pure, so the patient typically wants to be viewing through the center to obtain the best possible, unaltered vision. Knowing where the optical centers are on a lens also helps you determine the *distance between optical centers* (DBOC) of the glasses. The DBOC of a pair of glasses typically should be the same as a patient's *interpupillary distance* (PD), the distance between their pupils in a far gaze. Therefore, when dispensing glasses to patients, you will want to mark the optical centers on their new glasses to ensure that they are looking through the optical center of the lens. Future chapters will discuss how incorrectly placed optical centers cause problems and how to measure the patient's PD. For now, we will describe how to find the optical centers and the DBOC of a pair of glasses using a lensometer.

By definition, the optical center of the lens is "that part of the lens through which a ray of light passes when its path both before and after refraction by the lens are in the same direction." This definition is from the Dictionary of Visual Science. What this means is that the image path entering the lens will be parallel to that exiting the lens. There is no refracting of images through this point on the lens.

Why, then, do we want the patient to look through this point? Doesn't this mean that the patient will not appreciate any of the power in a lens? Let's look again at how a lens refracts light. You will notice that the rays of light that enter through the very center of the lens do not undergo any refraction; only the peripheral rays do.

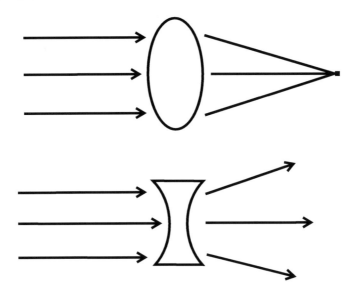

Central rays through the lens do not refract. Only peripheral rays refract.

As you can see, if we were to eliminate all the peripheral rays transmitted through the lens, it would not matter where the retina was located because the central ray would always provide a clear single point of focus on the retina. It is the peripheral rays that contribute to the varying focal distances from a lens.

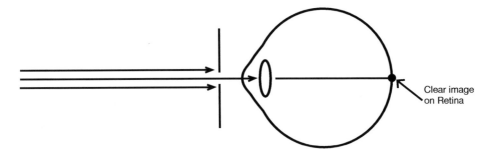

Light through a pinhole allows only central rays through

It is therefore not the central image rays, but rather the peripheral rays, that refract to give a lens its power. You can test this yourself if you are someone who typically needs glasses to see clearly. Take off your glasses and look at some distant object. Probably quite blurry. Now punch a very small pin-sized hole through a piece of paper and look through the hole at the same object. This has made the object clearer even though you do not have your glasses on. Why? Because you have eliminated the peripheral rays and are seeing the object only with the central rays. The central rays are falling upon the retina without the peripheral rays adding a focal point either behind or in front of the retina. This is commonly called the "pinhole effect."

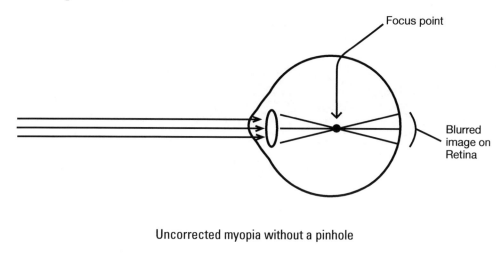

Uncorrected myopia without a pinhole

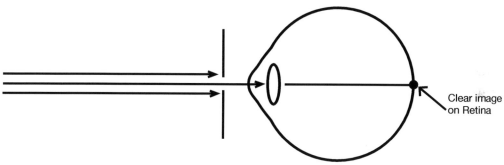

Uncorrected myopia with a pinhole

As we can now see, if a patient were to look through the lens at any point other than the optical center, the patient would experience an image different from the one intended by the prescription in the lens.

There are times when you do not want the patient to look through the optical center of a lens, such as if the patient has an eye-turn, also called *strabismus.* By displacing the optical center, you induce *prism* that will redirect image rays to where the macula is actually located. This will be a topic of a future chapter, but for now, we will be content simply to learn how to find the optical center of a lens using the lensometer.

To find the optical centers:

1. Place the lens into the lensometer as if you were to read the power.
2. While looking into the eyepiece, turn the power drum until the

intersection of the mires is visible. They will not likely both become clear at the same time due to any cylinder correction in the lens, as we saw in the previous section. But as long as you can visualize the intersection, you will be able to proceed.

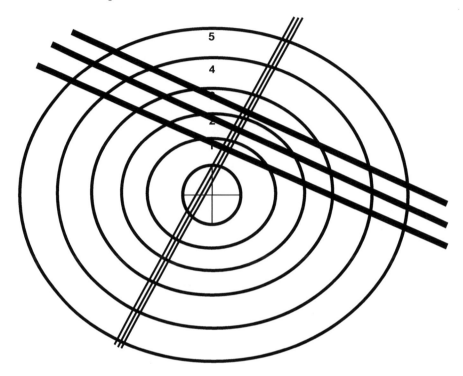

3. Move the eyeglasses by hand until the intersection of the mires is in the center of the reticle grid.

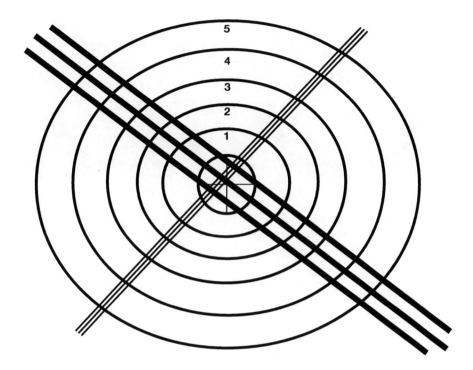

4. With the ink marker attachment, press the marker onto the lens. Be sure you dip the marker into the inkwell first.

5. The glasses will now have three ink marks in a horizontal line. The center mark is the location of the optical center of the lens.

6. Repeat the procedure with the other lens.

With this information, you now can measure the distance between optical centers (DBOC) of the glasses. Again, this measurement should typically be the same as the patient's PD.

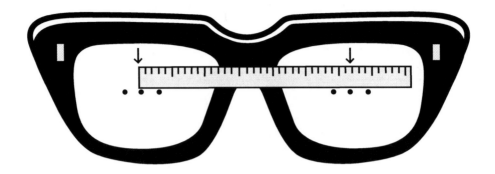

The distance between optical centers (DBOC) is the distance
between center ink marks.

Place the "0" mark on the center ink spot on one of the lenses. The DBOC is
the measurement that corresponds to the center ink spot on the other lens.

Base Curve Measurements

The base curve is an important part of the lens analysis workup. Oftentimes,
when a patient makes a vague complaint such as, "These glasses just don't feel
right," a change in the base curve relative to the patient's old glasses is often the
culprit. Yet many times the base curve is overlooked by the beginner optician, and
even by experienced opticians, as a possible cause.

What is the base curve? It is the curvature, measured in *diopters*, of the front
surface of the lens. (Very old lenses were made with the base curve on the back
surface, but you are not likely to run across any of these except for maybe in an
antique store.) The higher the base curve, the steeper or more curved the lens
will be. The lower the base curve, the flatter the lens will be. From the patient
perspective, the higher/steeper the base curve, the more magnified things may
appear.

The base curve is measured with a device called the *lens clock*. This is used by
placing its three pegs perpendicular to the lens surface and reading the black
number corresponding to the dial pointer.

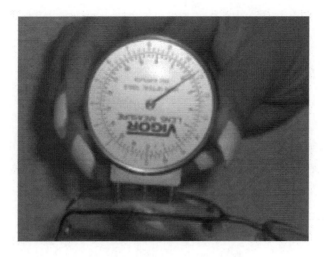

The optical lab that makes the lenses usually sets certain prescription ranges with the same base curve. For example, all lenses in the range of -1.00D to -3.00D will have the same base curve, all lenses -3.00D to -5.00D will have the same base curve, and so forth. This may create adaptation difficulties for patients who just barely fell into one category with their previous glasses, and whose prescription change pushed them into the next category with their new glasses. This change in base curve may give the patient a nauseous feeling resulting from the perceived magnification difference. Typically, the patient will adapt within a couple of weeks. But,if you recognize that a base curve change was made, you are better able to explain the patient's symptoms to them. If the patient is unable to adapt, you are typically able to make a special request to the lab to make a prescription in a base curve outside its normal range.

Detecting lens warpage with the lens clock

Unless the lens is aspheric, the front surface should be spherical. (We will discuss aspheric lenses in a future chapter. It is a lens specially cut to be thin and lightweight, usually for those needing high-power lenses). Spherical means the lens clock should give the same reading whether you "clock" the lens in the vertical or horizontal axis. If there is a difference, and you are sure the lens in not aspheric, then you have a warped lens. One exception to this is in some new thinner and lighter lens material, called high index lenses, which may have a slight base curve difference in the vertical and horizontal axes.

Modern lenses are more prone to warpage than the glass lenses of years ago. So if a patient complains that their glasses "just aren't right," a check for base curve warpage should be part of your analysis. A lens analysis worksheet in the final chapter should guide you through most cases of patients complaining about their new glasses. Have these copied and ready for your use.

Common case involving base curve changes

Oftentimes, after cataract surgery, patients' prescriptions will change dramatically. This may put the patients into lenses with base curves they have not had before. Although these patients may report their vision as clearer than ever, they feel sick every time they put the glasses on. Base curve measurements are very important in these cases, as the dramatic change in power likely led to a change in the base curve.

Measuring Prism

There is an old adage that "prism is poison." Although this may be a little harsh when applied to those patients who genuinely need the help prism provides, it also can be the cause of many headaches for the optician when it is present in glasses when it should not be.

First, let us describe what prism is and what it is not. Prism is not a thing; it is not something you can see in glasses and not something you can "go fetch" from the lab. What it is, in its most basic element, is the effect observed when one side of a lens is ground thicker then the other side. The thin side is called the *apex* and the thick side is called the *base*. It is measured in *prism diopters*. One prism diopter will displace an image 1 cm at a distance of 1 meter, two prism diopters will displace an image 2 cm at a distance of 1 meter, and so forth.

What this creates, then, is a displacement of the image viewed through the lens. The greater the difference in thickness between the two sides of the lens, the greater the prism power, and therefore the greater the image displacement. The object being viewed through a prism will always be displaced in the direction of the apex. This is because light will always bend toward the base. Here is an illustration of what happens when an image is passed through a prism lens.

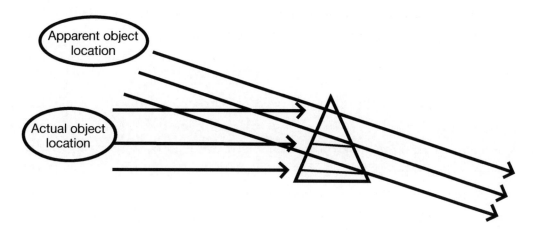

Prism redirecting an image. The apparent object location is found
by following the resultant rays back to their "apparent" source.

So when is prism used in glasses? It is not uncommon for a patient to have one
eye turned slightly in, out, up, or down, relative to the other eye. You have likely
seen a person like this and not been quite sure which eye is the one looking at
you! Without prism, this person would likely see double, since each eye is looking
in a different direction. Prism, with its ability to redirect images, is ground into
the lenses to help the person see a single image. Prism does not straighten the
eye, however; it simply redirects the image to where the eye is pointed.

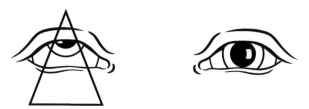

Schematic illustration of prism in glasses for an eye turn

A simple way to remember which way the prism should be directed for a given
eye turn is to think of prism as an arrow, with the apex being the tip and the
base being the tail. The arrow tip should point in the direction of the eye turn.
The doctor will do all the work in determining the amount of the prism and its
direction. This will be on the prescription form. Prism is always spoken of *in the
direction of the base,* so if an eye is turned upward (as in our illustration above), the
prism over that eye would be referred to as *base down. Base out* would mean the eye
was turned inward, and so forth.

The amount of prism is usually split between the two lenses to avoid one lens from becoming exceedingly thick. Usually the doctor will have the prescription written with the prism amount already split between the two lenses. But in case it isn't, let's look at how to do it and why it can be done.

We must remember that prism is used to correct a *relative* difference in the way the two eyes are pointed. In other words, if the left eye is pointed **down** and the right eye is straight ahead, then the right eye is also pointed **up** *relative* to the left eye. The brain doesn't know which eye is "straight ahead," only that it is seeing double. The same goes for horizontal deviations. If the left eye is pointed **outward**, and the right eye is straight ahead, then the right eye is also pointed **outward** *relative* to the left.

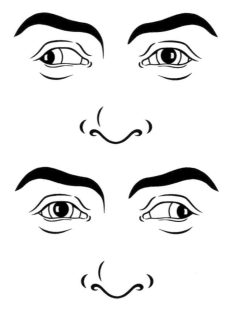

Horizontal eye turn

So how does this help us split the prism between the lenses in order to minimize lens thickness? Let's take an example of a patient whose right eye turns out 20 prism diopters, as seen in the illustration below. This patent is prescribed 20 prism diopters Base-in (BI) over the right eye. You may not have seen a lens with prism yet in your career, but 20 diopters of prism is one very thick lens! Grinding 20 diopters of prism into this patient's right lens would be cosmetically poor and cause the patient to walk with a tilt from the weight! However, if we remember to think of eye turns as a *relative difference* between the two eyes and not pay attention only to the eye with the turn, we would see that the patient has a total 20 prism diopter difference between the two eyes, outward from each other. Therefore, 20 prism diopters Base-in over the right eye is the same as 10 prism diopters Base-in over each eye, to give a total of 20 diopters Base-in. Ten diopters of prism is still thick, but both lenses will be equally thick and a lot more cosmetically appealing than 20 diopters all over one eye.

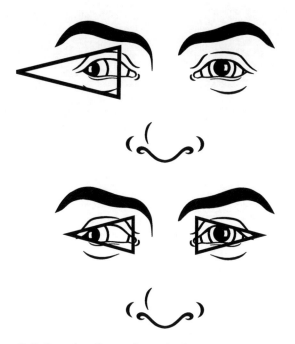

Splitting prism (bottom) over both eyes creates cosmetically
more attractive glasses by reducing lens thickness.

Let's look at a vertical deviation now. Suppose a patient has a six-prism diopter upward turn of the right eye and is prescribed 6-prism diopters base down over the right eye, as in the illustration below. This would work to solve the patient's problem, but it would not be very cosmetically appealing. The bottom of the right lens would be much thicker then the bottom of the left lens. So we would want to split the prism between the two lenses. This patient has a *relative* difference of 6-prism diopters vertically between the two eyes, with the right eye relatively pointed up and the left eye relatively pointed down. If we give this patient 3-prism diopters base down over the right eye and 3 prism diopters base up over the left eye, this is the same as an entire 6-prism diopters base up over the left, but much more cosmetically pleasing.

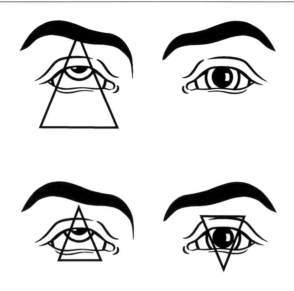

Both examples have the same net effect, but splitting the prism reduces lens thickness.

As a double check when calculating how much prism a patient will appreciate when splitting prism between two lenses, it is important to remember that the prism is *additive in the horizontal axis*, but measured as a *difference in the vertical*, as seen in these last two examples. Putting 10 BO prism over each eye gives a total of a 20 BO effect (*add* the BOs); putting 3 BD over the right eye and 3 BU over the left gives a total of 6 BU over the left eye (the total difference between 3 BU and 3 BD). Similarly, 10 BO over one eye and 10 BI over the other eye have a zero net effect (like adding the same number of opposite signs). It just moves the image for both eyes off to the side, but an equal distance. 3 BU over both eyes also has zero net effect (there is no difference between 3 BU and 3 BU); it just moves the image for both eyes downward equally. Granted, in each of these cases where there is no net prism effect, the patient would have a skewed perception of reality, since images straight ahead would look off-center. But neither case would solve any relative difference in eye position or prevent a person from seeing double.

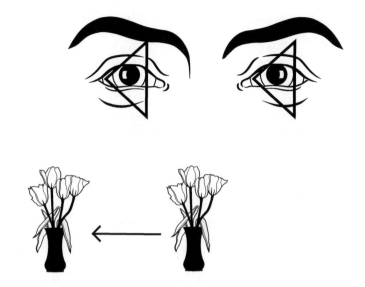

Prism of the same amount and in the same orientation over each eye
will displace the image in the direction of the prism's apex.

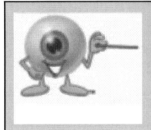 **Focus Point:** When calculating the total prism in a pair of glasses, horizontal prism is additive, and vertical prism is calculated as a difference.

So let's say a patient is picking up his or her glasses with prescribed prism, and you wish to make sure the lab ground in the correct amount of prism for the patient. How do you check this? First, we must know the three ways prism can be defined clinically.

1. Prescribed prism: This is the amount of prism prescribed by the doctor.
2. Measured prism: This is the amount of prism ground into the lens by the laboratory.
3. Effective prism: This is the actual prism the patient is experiencing.

Prescribed prism may be different from measured prism if the lab makes an error in manufacturing the lenses. Effective prism may be different from prescribed prism if you, the optician, make an incorrect PD measurement (we will discuss how this happens shortly). As we can see, from a clinical perspective, effective prism must be checked and compared to prescribed prism to make sure the patient is getting the prism he or she needs.

In order to measure effective prism:

1. Place the glasses on the patient and have a wet-erase Sharpie pen in your hand.
2. Sit directly in front of the patient and have him or her look straight at your left eye. With the marker, place a mark on the lens over the patient's right pupil. This mark is identifying the patient's visual axis.
3. Do the same with the other eye. Have the patient look at your right eye and place a mark on the lens over the patient's left eye.

   By having the patient look at you eye to eye, you are best able to measure the location of his or her pupil in a distance gaze position while minimizing the effects of *parallax* (the errors in perception that arise from viewing an object off-axis).

4. Place the glasses in the lensometer, with the pen mark centered over the lens stop, and read the prism amount from the lensometer grid.

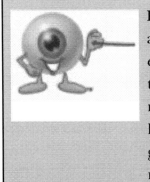

Focus Point: Measuring *effective prism* is the only way to accurately measure the amount of prism the patient is experiencing. The *only* way to measure effective prism is to have the patient sitting in front of you so that you can mark his or her visual axis, centering these marks into the lensometer and reading the prism from the lensometer grid. You may learn shortcuts from other opticians, but do not be fooled. There are no shortcuts. You must take the time to mark the patient's visual axis through the lenses.

Looking at your newly marked lens in the lensometer, you will want to keep in mind that each ring of the lensometer grid is one prism diopter in most cases, except for the first ring, which typically represents 0.5 prism diopters. If the lens mires intersect higher than the grid center, you have base-up prism. If the mire intersection is lower than the grid center, you have base-down prism. For horizontal prism readings, you must be aware of which lens you are measuring, the right or the left. For example, if you have the right lens in the lensometer and the mires are offset to the left of the center of the grid, then you have *Base-out* prism. If, however, you have the left lens in the lensometer and the mires are offset to the left, you have *Base-in* prism. Remember, base in and out refer to whether the prism base is closer to the nose or the ear respectively, so you must be aware of which lens you are measuring to know which direction the prism base is in.

Let's look at a couple of examples.

After dotting the visual axis of a left lens, place the lens in a lensometer, centering your dot. You'll see this:

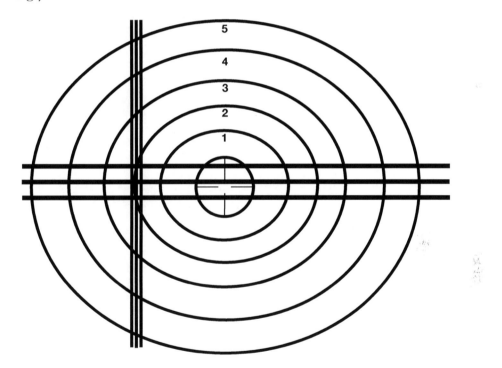

What is the amount of effective prism in this lens? Let's look at where the intersection of the mires line up on the grid and break it down into its horizontal and vertical components.

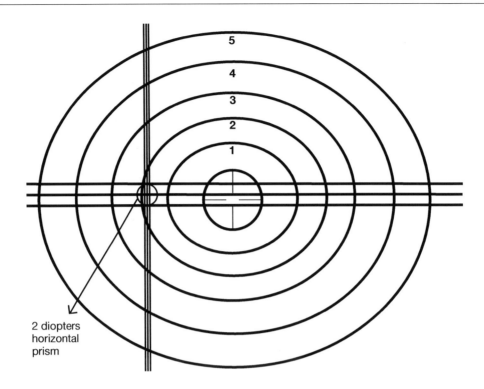

2 diopters
horizontal
prism

Let's look for any horizontal prism first. To do so, look at where the mire intersection sits on the grid's horizontal axis. In this case, the intersection is on the 2-diopter ring on the grid's horizontal axis. Therefore, we have 2 diopters of horizontal prism. But in what direction? If this is a left lens, then the intersection is toward the nasal side of the lens, and therefore is Base-in prism.

Now let's look for any vertical prism. The mires sit directly on the horizontal axis and there is no deviation into the vertical axis. Therefore, there is no vertical prism in this lens.

Here's another more complicated example. You have a left lens dotted and sitting in the lensometer with this view:

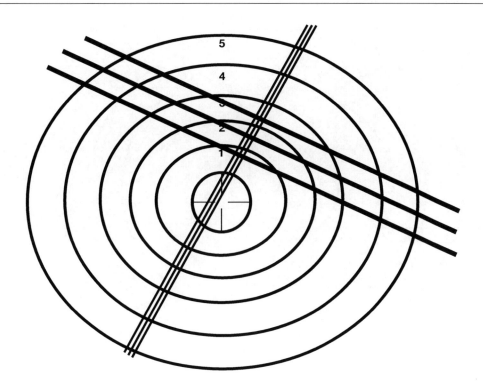

How much prism is in this lens?

   This lens has what is called compound prism, meaning both a vertical and horizontal prism. We can see that the intersection of the mires is offset both vertically and horizontally from the center of the grid. In cases such as this, it can sometimes be difficult for the novice to understand how to read the prism, because the intersection is diagonal from the center of the grid. *Remember: You must read the prism only from the horizontal and vertical grid axis.* So how do we do this when the mires' intersection is diagonal to the center of the grid? By visualizing a box with two opposite corners lying at the grid center and the mires' intersection. In doing so, the other two corners of your imaginary box will be your horizontal and vertical prism measurements.

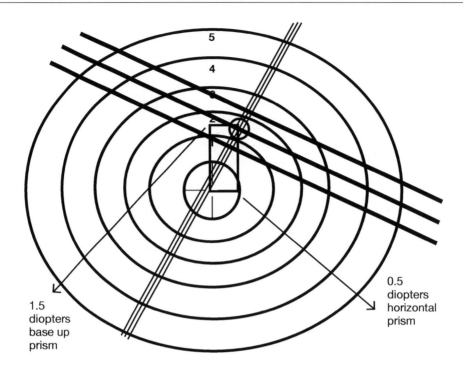

In this example, we see that the intersection of the mires lies 1.5 prism diopters up from center on the vertical axis and 0.5 prism diopters right of center on the horizontal axis. If this is the left lens, what direction is the prism base? Vertical prism is always as it appears on the grid regardless of the lens being tested. Up is up and down is down no matter which lens you have. So we have 1.5 diopters of prism Base-up in this lens. Being the left lens, the intersection of the mires will lie on the temporal (ear) side of the lens; therefore, we have 0.5 prism diopters Base-out.

This lens would therefore be recorded as 1.5Δ BU and 0.5ΔBO OS.

Now let's look at examples of how to combine the values you find for each eye to arrive at the total prism a patient has in his or her glasses.

Example 1:

In the lensometer, you measure 2 BU in the right eye and 3 BD in the left. What is the total amount of prism the patient will experience through these glasses?

Remember that when measuring vertical prism, to find the total amount you must calculate the *difference* between the two lenses. In this case, the difference between 2BU and 3 BD is 5 diopters of vertical prism. Whether you call this 5 BU in the right eye or 5 BD in the left, both ways of writing this says the same thing.

Example 2:

In the lensometer, you measure 3 BO in the left eye and 3 BO in the right. What total amount of prism will the patient experience through these glasses?

Remember that with horizontal prism, the prism is *additive*; therefore, 3 BO in each eye will give the patient a total of 6 BO (3+3). If, on the other hand, the lenses had 3 BO in the left and 3 BI in the right, the net effect would be 0 prism. This would be the same as adding a +3 to a -3 to arrive at zero.

Prentice Rule

The following equation, called the *Prentice Rule,* will help you understand how glasses made with an incorrect PD (inter-pupillary distance) can induce unwanted prism or cause the patient not to experience the proper amount of prism they need. You may recall that there were only two equations in this entire book that were important to remember. The first was the relationship between the power of a lens (diopters) and the focal point of the lens. This is the second. The equation is this:

Prism = F × d

F is the power of the lens (in diopters), and *d* is the decentration of the optical center (in centimeters) away from the patient's pupil. As you can see from the equation, having the optical center of any lens decentered from what is the patient's true PD can induce unwanted prism and, therefore, headaches and double vision for the patient! This equation also tells you that the higher the power of the lens, the more exacting the PD measure must be, as even a small decentration of a high-power lens can induce problematic prism. Typically, patients are able to tolerate about 0.5 diopter of unwanted vertical prism and 3–4 diopters of unwanted horizontal prism before symptoms begin to occur.

The purpose of learning this equation is to help you understand that especially for higher-power lenses, a small misstep in measuring the patient's inter-pupillary distance can result in a large amount of prism (and all the side effects) unintentionally given to the patient.

Remember, both the power of the lens (F) and the amount of prism are measured in units of *diopters*. It can be confusing having two completely different aspects of a lens using the same notation.

Here's an example:

A prescription of +5.00 DS OU is made for a patient. The patient's PD is 64mm. The distance between optical centers of the lenses, however, comes back from the lab at 72mm. This is a 0.8 cm (8mm) total decentration. Using the equation *Prism = F × d*, where the power of the lens is +5.00 diopters and the decentration, *d*, is 0.8, we arrive at 4 diopters of prism.

Prism = 5 × 0.8 = 4

Four diopters of prism is likely going to be enough to create some unpleasing symptoms in this patient. Now, is this prism Base-out or Base-in?

To answer this question, we need to think in terms of the shape of the lens and how it is positioned relative to the patient's pupils. Recall that a plus-power lens has a thicker center than edge and a minus-power lens has a thicker edge than center. Therefore, prescription lenses can be thought of schematically as two prisms side by side, either with bases or apexes touching.

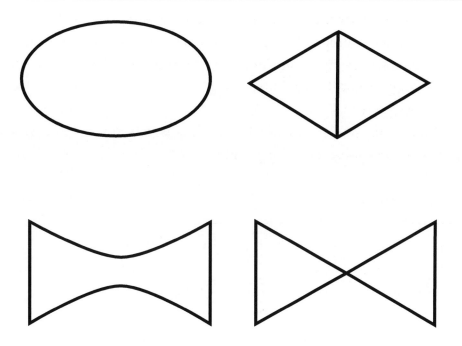

Top: The plus-power lens is thicker in the center.
Bottom: The minus-power lens is thicker on the edge.

In our example, we have plus-power lenses (+5.00) spaced further apart than the patient's eyes (patient's PD is 64mm, but the optical centers of the lenses are spaced apart 72mm). To determine the direction of the prism this will create, it is easiest to visualize this scenario on the patient.

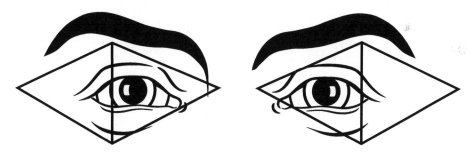

Plus lenses placed on a patient with a distance between optical centers greater than the patient's PD

As we can see from this example, if the distance between optical centers is greater than the patient's own PD and we have plus-power lenses, then the prism base (the thickest part of the lens) will be outward relative to the pupils. Therefore, in this example, we have created 4 Base-out prism for this patient.

This was an overly simplified example, because patients rarely have the same prescription in each eye. To be the most exact, you should apply this equation to each eye individually.

Let's look at an example in which each lens is of a different power and we must calculate the prism for each eye individually.

A prescription of -5.00 DS OD and -6.00 DS OS is prescribed (recall OD is the right eye and OS is the left eye). The right lens is decentered 4mm outwardly from the pupil, and the left lens is decentered 5mm outwardly from the pupil. What is the amount of prism induced and in what direction?

$$\text{Right eye: Prism} = 5 \times 0.4 = 2 \text{ diopters}$$
$$\text{Left eye:} \quad \text{Prism} = 6 \times 0.5 = 3 \text{ diopters}$$

In what direction is this prism induced? Let's again visualize it on a patient.

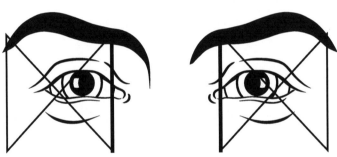

A minus lens decentered outward on a patient

As we can see when we visualize where the thick (base) and thin (apex) part of the lens falls when we decenter a minus-power lens outwardly, the thick part of the lens will lie toward the nose of the patient for each eye. This creates Base-in prism.

Therefore, we have created a total of 5 diopters Base-in prism. (Recall that the horizontal prism is *additive.* 2 BI + 3BI = 5BI.)

This also is slightly oversimplified, as nearly all prescriptions will have some astigmatic correction. You may recall from our discussion on prescriptions that astigmatism means one axis will have a different power from the other, and by looking at the prescription, you can determine the power in each axis. You can also calculate the unwanted prism induced in each axis in a decentered lens by using the *Prentice Rule* equation for each axis individually.

This equation may also be used to calculate induced vertical prism if you should find that the patient's pupil is actually sitting above or below the optical center of the lens.

The point here is not to have you calculate the induced prism on each case of a decentered lens you run across. Rather, it's to help you appreciate that prism can be unintentionally induced in a lens by a poor PD measurement. Also, keep in mind that this equation illustrates that the higher the power of the lens, the greater impact having an erroneous PD measurement will be. So if a patient with new glasses complains about seeing double or experiencing dizziness or headaches, you will want to check for unwanted prism by marking the patient's pupil location on the lens and checking for prism in a lensometer.

Measuring Progressives

Progressive addition lenses (PAL) permit the patient to see distant, intermediate, and near objects all with one lens and all without any lines. What's the catch? These lenses are optically far more sensitive to slight misalignments than any other lens. Therefore, not only must great care be taken when fitting these lenses for a patient (we will discuss this in a future chapter), but great care must be taken also when measuring the power of a progressive in a lensometer.

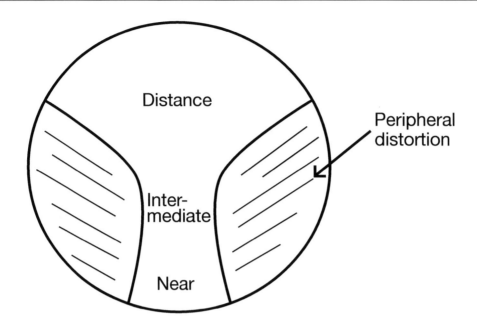

Illustration of optical areas in progressive lens

In order to have all the powers (distance, intermediate, and reading) blend without a line, some distortion is always going to be present in the peripheral part of the lens.

When measuring the power of a PAL, therefore, be sure you know where you are on the lens and where each of the three powers is supposed to be located. Fortunately, PAL manufacturers have made this easy for us with the use of a template. There are hundreds of different brands of progressive lenses, and each one will have a slightly different template. Your office likely will use only a few brands of progressives, so you will not have to hunt all day for the template appropriate for the lens you are working with.

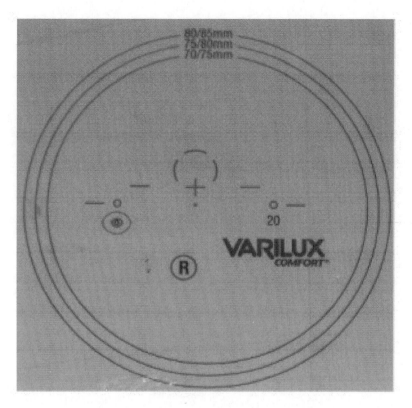

Example of a progressive template (courtesy Essilor)

Before you can use the template to measure the power of your lens, you must know which brand of PAL you are working with to ensure you use the right template. Etched into every progressive lens is a faint trademark characteristic to that particular brand. Again, your office will likely use only a few types of progressives, so you will become adept very quickly at recognizing the symbol. However, until then, you will be using a book call the *Progressive Identifier* that has a diagram of all the possible markings you may find. Use it to match the trademark symbol you find etched on the lens to determine the brand of PAL you are dealing with.

Finding the etched trademark will sometimes turn you into a contortionist. The lighting on the lens must be just right. Some patients with too much time on their hands may come across it and complain that their lenses are scratched. To help you find the mark, most optical offices have an instrument called the PAL Identifier, which includes a green backlight and a magnifier.

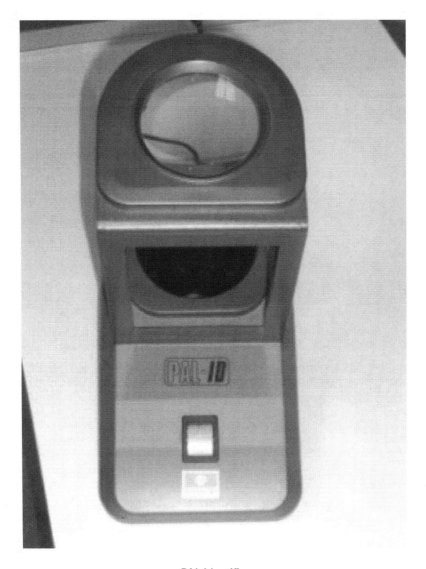

PAL Identifier

The template will have the same trademark symbol you found etched on the lenses. This way you know you are using the right template.

In addition to the etched trademark, there will be a circular etch mark on both sides of the lenses. Mark them with a Sharpie pen, because the etch marks will help you line up the lens on the template.

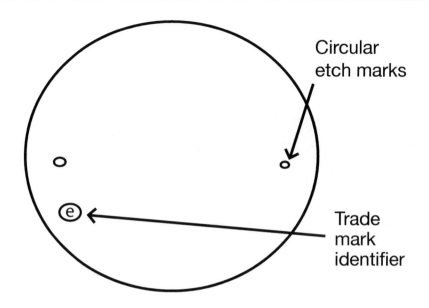

Illustration of etch marking seen on a progressive lens

Place the lens onto the template with your marked circular etch marks aligned with the circular marks on the template. The template will now give you a visual representation of the optics involved with the lens. With your Sharpie pen, trace the template directly onto the lens.

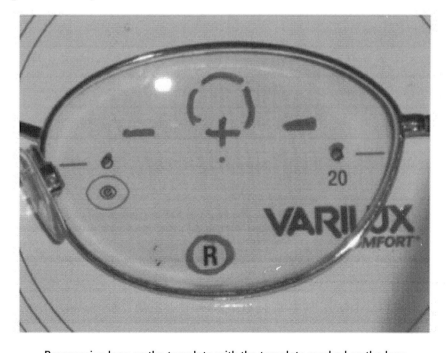

Progressive lens on the template with the template marked on the lens

Once the template has been transferred to the lens, this is what your lens will look like:

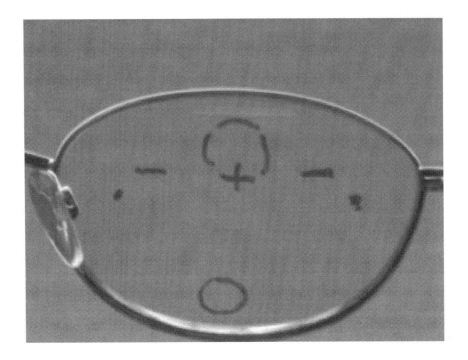

You will notice the following locations on the template you have just transferred:

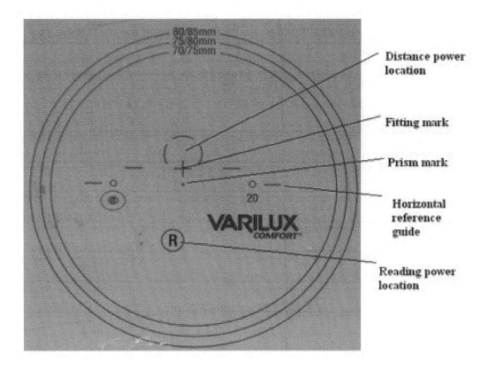

Various parts of the progressive template

1. The distance location. Set this mark in the lensometer to measure the power in the distance portion of the lens.
2. The prism mark. Set this point in the lensometer to measure the amount of prism in the lenses.
3. The fitting mark. When you dispense the lenses, this mark should sit at the same location as the pupil of the patient's eyes.
4. The reading location. Set this mark in the lensometer to measure the reading power of the lens. (As with a line bifocal, the difference between this power and the distance power is the *Add* power). Add power is often etched onto the lens as well as in the temporal region.
5. The horizontal reference guide. These lines should be horizontal to the floor when the glasses are on the patient.

Place the marked lens on the patient to ensure the patient is looking through the distance location of the lens and has ample reading area, and make any adjustments necessary to center the marks appropriately.

Using the templates will greatly simplify your measurements of PALs. With the template, you can do a complete analysis of the lens powers and confirm the proper fitting height of the glasses on the patient's face. The fitting mark confirmation is essential when dispensing the lenses due to the nature of the PAL design. If that mark is slightly off horizontally, the patient could be forced to look through the peripheral distortion areas of the lens. If the fitting mark is slightly too high, the patient would be forced to look through the intermediate power when looking straight ahead and therefore have blurry distance vision. Other types of lens design, such as single-vision glasses or bifocals, may allow you a little fudge room in the way the lens sits on the patient's face, but the PAL is not one of those! The details make all the difference when measuring and dispensing a PAL

Chapter 2 Test

1. With a pair of glasses supplied by your manager, analyze the prescription using the test sheet on the following page.

2. A patient complains of seeing double with his new glasses. Describe the steps needed to determine the amount of prism, if any, the patient is experiencing.

3. A patient's PD is 62. She has a prescription of -5.00 DS in the right eye and -7.00DS in the left. The optical centers are displaced 3mm outward in each eye. How much prism and in what direction has been induced by this error?

4. How would you detect warpage in a lens?

5. Approximately what add power would you expect to see on the prescription of a 50-year-old?

6. Before measuring the power of a progressive, what must you know first?

7. What is the name of the instrument used to measure the base curve of a lens?

8. What is the fitting mark on the PAL template used for?

Eyeglass Prescription Analysis Test

	Sphere	Cylinder	Axis	Prism	Base
OD					

Distance:

OS					

	Power	Seg height	Seg width
OD			

Add:

OS			

Base Curve OD: Base curve OS:

Warpage?

DBOC:

DBS:

CHAPTER 3

Frame Selection

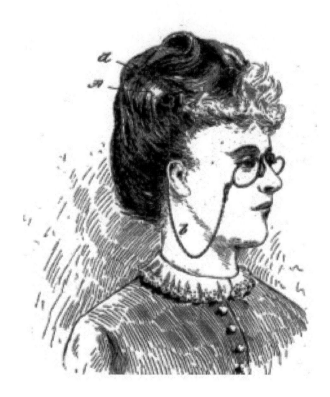

FRAMES come in many sizes and shapes. This is a good thing, since heads come in many sizes and shapes. However, not every frame is proper for every prescription. Selecting the proper frame is essential in creating an acceptable final product. Patients will inevitably experience a gravitational pull toward the glasses that are the least appropriate for them. Your job is to save them from themselves and steer them in a direction that will make both the patient, and, if they are married, their spouse, happy.

There are two things to look at when guiding a patient through the frame selection process: the patient's prescription and the patient's face. Placing a high prescription into a large frame, for example, would result in an unacceptably heavy and thick pair of glasses. Certain facial characteristics, such as a large nose, can become less noticeable with the proper selection of frames. This chapter will discuss what types of frames to use (and which ones to avoid) when fitting a patient with glasses.

Before doctors can work with a broken bone, they must first know the name of the bone that is broken and how it interacts with surrounding bones. Similarly, before discussing the proper selection of a frame for a patient's face, we must first know the basic components of a pair of frames. This will come in handy when we discuss frame adjustments in the next chapter, so be sure you understand the basic parts of a frame before continuing beyond this chapter.

Frame Parts

Here are the basics of frame anatomy:

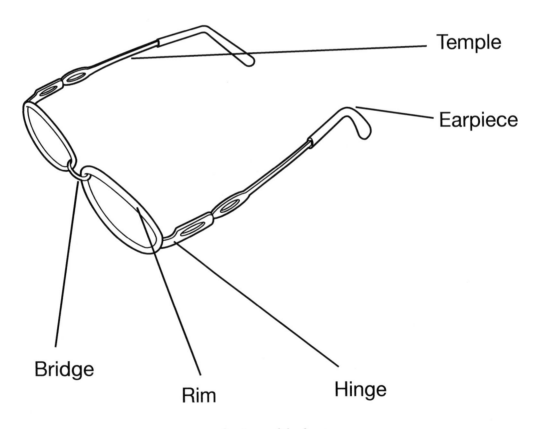

Anatomy of the frame

Frame: The entire "skeleton" of the glasses. Everything that goes into holding the lenses in place and the eyeglasses on the face. Just like the skull, leg bones and spine all make up a person's skeleton; the frame is the entirety of its parts.

Temples: Support the frame around the ears.

Hinges: Connect the temples to the rim.

Rim: The part of the frame that holds the prescription lenses in place.

Rim Groove: Groove on the inside of the rim that helps support the lens.

Bridge: Holds the two rims together.

Nosepads: Distributes the weight of the frame and lenses evenly across the nose.

Frame Materials

There are many frame materials from which to chose. Typically, patients select a style of frame they like, unaware that the material of the frame may not suit their lifestyle. This is where your expertise comes in. Knowing the benefits of the frame materials along with asking detailed questions about the patient's lifestyle will make a harmonious blend of form and function.

The key features you want to look for in a frame are:

1. Its ability to be adjusted easily and hold its shape
2. Its material composition—will it cause an allergic skin reaction in some patients?
3. Its weight
4. Its cost

Plastic Frames

1. Zyl

   Zyl (Cellulose Acetate) is among the most common types of material seen in plastic frames today for several reasons. Zyl is inexpensive compared to other materials it is easy to work with, and it comes in nearly any color.

Zyl does not come without its pitfalls, however. Although Zyl is easily adjusted, it tends to become brittle with age. Additionally, you can typically identify this material by the white grainy film it leaves on the surface of the frame after several months or years of wear. This film is created by the patient's sweat, drawing *plasticizers* (elements of Zyl that keep it pliable) out of the material which then deposit on the surface. Zyl also burns easily, and heat can loosen the hinges. For this reason, try to make your adjustments with a minimal use of heat.

2. Optyl

Optyl weighs less than Zyl and does not use plasticizers, so no white film deposits on the frame. The main benefit to Optyl is that it is considered hypoallergenic, meaning very few people will experience an allergic reaction from its contact with the skin.

Optyl heats well without becoming damaged, and temples can be heated and lengthened with gentle stretching. However, Optyl does not hold its adjustments as well as Zyl, and over time it can return somewhat to its original shape. As with Zyl, Optyl can become brittle with age.

Metal frames

1. Nickel

Nickel is the most common metal frame material you will see, primarily because of its relatively low cost and its ability to hold its shape well once adjusted.

The main drawback to nickel is its allergy-causing properties. Patients will come into your office complaining that the temples on their glasses and the surrounding skin have turned green. The patients' sweat breaks down the nickel and turns it as green as a cheap ring.

These frames are good for those on a tight budget who do not like the look of plastic frames.

2. Titanium

Titanium frames are ultra lightweight and hypoallergenic (they will not turn green). As you can imagine, patients have to pay considerably more for these benefits.

This material is usually best matched with a premium lens, which will further reduce the weight, or it is used for those patients with a history of green temples from previous nickel frames.

3. Memory metal

Memory metal is a combination of nickel and titanium. It is designed to be very durable and holds up well after twisting and bending. This property makes it ideal for parents with small children as well as active children who are rough with their frames.

Selecting a frame that fits well off the shelf is important with memory metals, because they do not maintain adjustments very well. Although small adjustments are possible, the frame generally returns to its pre-adjustment shape.

Memory metal frames are expensive, but they are well worth it for people who are tired of always having their frames adjusted.

Summary of Common Frame materials

PLASTICS	Pros	Cons
Zyl	Inexpensive	Not hypoallergenic
		Brittle with age
Optyl	Inexpensive	Slightly higher cost
	Easily adjusted	than Zyl
	Hypoallergenic	Brittle with age
METALS	Pros	Cons
Nickel	Inexpensive	Weight
	Easily adjusted	Not hypoallergenic
Titanium	Very lightweight and durable	Expensive
	Most hypoallergenic material	
Memory metal	Most flexible and durable	Adjustments not easy
	Lightweight	Expensive

Frames come in many other types of materials as well, but these are the most common.

Now we can resume our discussion on the proper frame selection.

Proper Frame for Prescription

The Myope

Nearsighted people have it fairly easy. There are not as many restrictions on this crowd as on hyperopes. At least for low prescriptions, if the frame fits well, you can use it. For higher prescriptions, however, keep some things in mind to make the finished pair of glasses look their best. For high minus prescriptions, remember the following:

1. *Keep the frame size small.*

The larger the frame, the thicker the edges of the lenses will be. Recall that for minus-power lenses, the edges are thicker than the center. This also means the further out from the center you go, the thicker the lens progressively becomes. So stay small on the frame size!

2. *The use of plastic frames will help hide edge thickness.*

A plastic frame will have a thicker border surrounding the lenses than metal or rimless frames. This trait of plastic frames can be used to help hide some of the edge thickness of a higher minus-power lens.

3. *Choose frames with rounded corners.*

Square corners on a frame will only accent the thickness of the edges. Try to steer the patient toward frames with rounded edges. Although a square frame may be in style, try to reserve the square frames only for those with low prescriptions.

The Hyperope

For farsighted patients, consider a couple of factors to create glasses the patient would be proud to wear. Hyperopic prescriptions lead to the infamous "Coke bottle" effect. In the section on lens options, we will discuss additional ways to minimize this effect with the proper use of lens materials, but for now we will limit our discussion to choosing the best frame.

1. *Keep the frame size small.*

The larger the frame, the thicker the center of the lens. Remember that for plus-power lenses, the center is thicker than the edges. So the larger the lens that must be cut to fit into a frame, the thicker the center will be relative to the edges of the lens.

2. *Only use frames with full rims.*

The thin edge of most plus-power lenses makes it impossible to cut a groove into it for the fishline support of a rimless frame. (A rimless frame uses a small string similar to a fishline to keep the lens supported in the frame.)

In order to make the edge thick enough to support this fishline, the center of the lens becomes much thicker than it otherwise would be. It is a good idea, therefore, to steer hyperopes away from rimless frames.

3. *Choose a frame with rounded corners.*

Just as the edge thickness in minus-power prescriptions will increase in a square frame, so will the center thickness of plus-power lenses with hyperopes. Reserve the square frames only for the mild prescriptions.

4. *Keep the vertex distance short.*

Vertex distance is the distance between the eye and the lens. The longer this distance, the greater the "bug-eyed" effect when looking at the patient's eyes. Select a frame with a short vertex distance and the patient's spouse will thank you!

The Presbyope

For patients over forty and in bifocals, trifocals, or progressives, there are two important things to remember. Bifocals and trifocals can be placed in almost any frame, but progressives cannot. Why is this? Think back to our previous chapter, where we defined these three types of multifocals. Bifocals and trifocals have their reading powers set in a separate *segment* that are ground onto the lens. This *seg* will always be set just below either the pupil (trifocal) or lower eyelid (bifocal). So although it is conceivable to select a frame that has a lower rim sitting directly below the pupil and therefore does not provide enough room for the bifocal or trifocal to fit, this is extremely rare. Even the narrowest frame, although it may cut off the bottom of the bifocal, will still be deep enough to allow the users to look under the bifocal seg line to some degree. As long as the wearers look under the seg line, they are getting their full reading power. Even in the rare case of an extremely narrow frame, seg heights on bifocals and trifocals are not set in stone. You could raise your seg height measurement on these types of lenses, and although the line may interfere with the patient's distance vision, you probably could get the line high enough for the patient to get some reading use out of the bifocal.

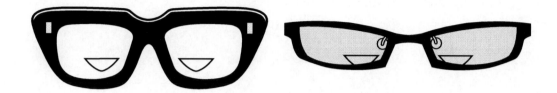

The large frame (left) provides more than ample depth for the entire bifocal. The small frame (right) cuts off the lower half of the bifocal, but still provides a sufficient, although small, reading area.

Progressive seg heights, unlike bifocals, are set in stone. The optics of a progressive lens are ground into the lens as part of the original manufacturing process. You cannot make the reading portion of the lens any higher or lower than it comes from the manufacturer. Too small a frame will cause the reading power in the lens to be lost completely when it is ground at the lab. The seg height you measure for bifocals and trifocals tells the optical lab where to set the seg line. The seg height you measure for progressives tells the lab where to set the *distance*. This means that if the frame is too narrow, the reading power may be lost. Exactly how to measure for these seg heights is the subject of the next chapter.

To better understand this, you need to know that lenses, of any type, are provided to the lab as *uncut* lenses. An "uncut" is a very large lens which already has the distance and reading powers ground into the lens. It is intentionally very large so the lab equipment can cut it down to the size and shape of the frame. A large frame might not require much lens cutting, while a small frame would.

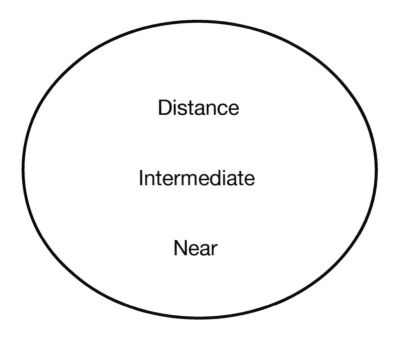

A progressive uncut lens with the location of the powers identified.

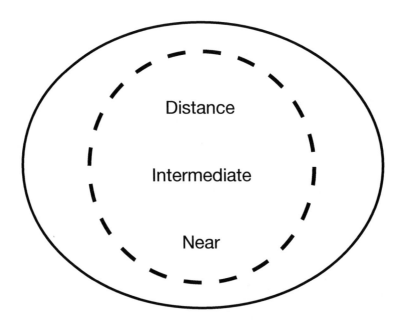

A progressive lens cut for a large frame (broken line).
Notice the near reading power is included in the cut.

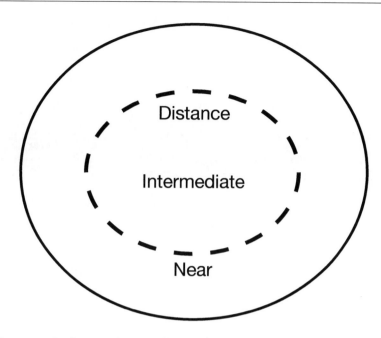

A progressive lens cut for a small frame (broken line). Notice that the near power
was sacrificed to get the lens to fit into a small frame.

Every brand of progressive has a different length between their distance
and reading levels. No one brand is ideal for every frame, and each has its own
pros and cons. Some progressives have a *short corridor* between the distance and
reading areas. Although this is the best type of progressive for small frames, it can
create additional peripheral distortions. The various types of progressives will be
discussed in the chapter on lens options, but for now be aware that progressives
and small frames typically are not friends of one another.

Proper frame for facial structure

Just as with clothing, not everyone will be able to get away with wearing the
same frame. Trying to appease patients by giving them what they want, when you
know it is not the best choice, will only create more problems for you down the
road. Sometimes it is best to tell a patient that a certain frame is just not right for
them. In this section, we will discuss how to select the best frame for the patient's
facial characteristics.

Face size and frame size

It is essential to select the proper frame size for the patient's face. Frames, like heads, come in different widths, lengths, and depths. The proper size frame will ensure the frame is comfortable for the patient.

The temple length:

The temple, the part of the frame that holds the glasses to the ear, ranges in length from 125mm to 150mm. For a frame in which the temples are sufficient to reach behind the ear to provide support, but not so long as to extend well past the ear, you must consider the depth of the patient's head—i.e., the eyes to the back of the ears.

Those with short depths should be steered toward frames with shorter temples (125–135mm); those with longer depths should be steered toward those with longer temples (140–150mm). The temple length will be marked on the inside of one of the temples.

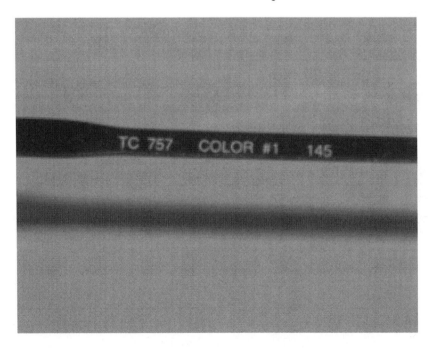

The temple length in this example is 145 (the number on the far right). The other notations refer to the frame model number and color. All three notations typically will appear together as in this example.

The bridge size:

Like head sizes, nose widths also vary by person. Fortunately, so do frame bridge widths. The bridge separates the two sides of the glasses and fits over the nose. Patients with narrow noses need a narrow bridge (16–18mm), while patients with a wider nose need a frame with a wider bridge (19–21mm). The bridge size will be the second of two numbers typically etched on the inward facing side of the bridge.

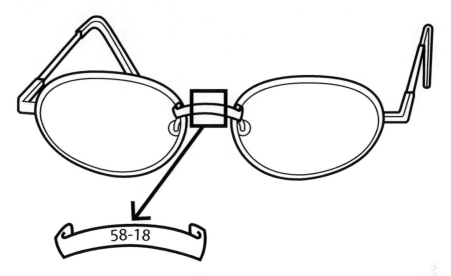

Bridge measurement location. The bridge size in this example is 18mm.

The frame size.

The frame size is composed of three measurements.

1. The A measurement. This is also called the *eyesize* and is the most common reference to frame size. *It is the longest horizontal length from one end of a rim to the other end of the same rim.* The A measurement is the first of two numbers typically etched on the inward facing side of the bridge, as seen in the illustration above. *The A measure, plus the bridge measure, is referred to as the Frame PD.* In general, it is a good idea to closely approximate this frame PD to the patient's PD, with the frame PD being only slightly larger. PD, if you recall, is an abbreviation for Pupillary Distance and refers to the distance between the patient's pupils. In the chapter on measuring a patient for glasses, we will learn how to measure this pupillary distance of a patient, both in distance gaze and reading gaze, and why this measurement is important when ordering a

pair of glasses. Frames obviously do not have pupils, and so calling any measurement of a frame a *PD* sounds more than a little silly; however, this is what the powers that be have done, so we must follow this definition of *Frame PD*.

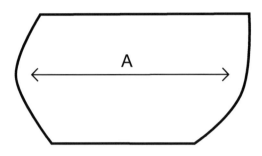

The A measurement

2. The B measure. This is the longest vertical length of the eyepiece.

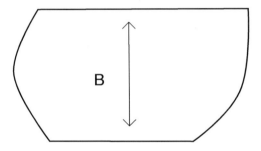

The B measurement

3. The ED measure. This is the longest diagonal measure of the eyepiece.

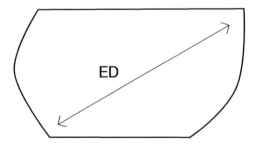

The ED measurement

You must take special care to correlate the frame size with the face size. Frames should not be too wide for the patient, or the temples will not fit snugly around the patient's ears.

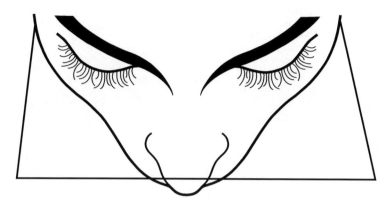

Frame too wide pinches in on temple region

Frames too narrow will put pressure on the temples on the side of the head.

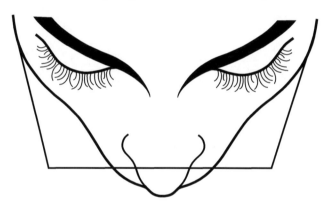

Frame too narrow will flair out at temple region

Facial forms

In general, the frame should help counter any prominent facial features. For example, if someone has an unusually large forehead, we would not want to put this person into a frame with a large and dark-colored superior rim, since this would draw attention upward toward the forehead. This patient is better served with a frame with a light-colored and thinner upper rim.

There are some general rules to keep in mind as we discuss each of the following face forms.

1. Horizontal lines widen.
2. Vertical lines elongate.
3. Curved lines soften.
4. Angular lines add definition.

Adding dark colors to any of the above lines accentuate the effect even further.

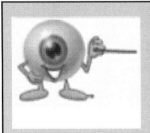 **Focus point:** Contrast the face shape to the frame shape. Angular faces need curvilinear frames. Curvilinear faces need angular frames.

1. Oval

   The oval face can look good in nearly any frame since there are no overbearing angles to the face. The frame should be as wide as the widest part of face.

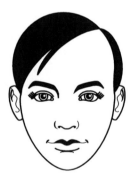

The oval face

2. Oblong

   This patient has a face that is longer than it is wide. In order to make the glasses look proportional on the head, select a frame which is a little deeper (longer from top to bottom) than average. Temples mounted low on the frame can help break the appearance of length. Frames with decorative or colored temples can help add width to the facial appearance.

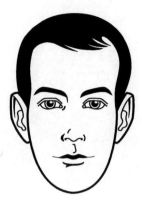

The oblong face

3. Square

For the patient with a square head (shorter and wider than average), select a frame with soft oval curves to help offset the angular head shape.

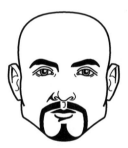

The square face

4. Round

For the round face, select a frame that is wider than deep. Additionally, if the prescription will allow for it, select a frame that has some distinctive sharp curves or angles to add contrast. Recall, however, that for high prescriptions you generally want to avoid frames with sharp edges and steer toward more rounded frames. Although a round pair of frames will draw attention to the round face, with higher prescriptions you will need to weigh priorities: the thickness of the lenses in a wide angular frame with the better cosmetic appearance of this type of frame on the face. There will not be one right answer in all situations.

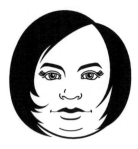

The round face

5. Base-up triangle

This patient has a wider forehead than chin. Try to avoid top-heavy frames, since this will only accentuate the size of the forehead region. Frames should be wider on the bottom with a low-mounted temple.

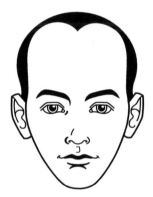

The Base-up face

6. Base-down triangle

The lower part of this patient's face is wider than the top. You may want to select a frame that has a heavy top rim to help the face appear more symmetrical. Temples should be mounted high on the frame. Frames that are rimless on the bottom half are a good choice as well.

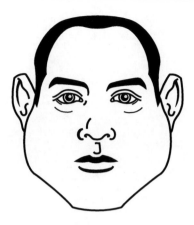

The Base-down face

7. Diamond

In this patient, the cheekbones are dramatic and pronounced. Avoid low-mounted temples. Lean toward frames with heavier upper rims to widen the forehead. Use frames with softer curves and colors.

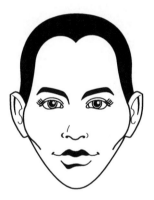

The diamond face

Summary of Face Shapes and Fitting Tips

FACE SHAPE	FITTING TIP
Oval	Nearly anything can look good!
Oblong (Longer than wide)	Deep frames. Low temple attachment. Decorative temples.
Round	Wider than deep. Angular.
Square	Soft curves. Avoid sharp angles.
Base-down triangle	Heavy top rim. Rimless on bottom of frame. Temples mounted high.
Base-up triangle	Avoid top-heavy frames. Temples mounted on bottom.
Diamond	Rounded frames. Soft colors. Avoid low-mounted temples.

Frame selection for children

Common sense reigns supreme when fitting a child with frames. Try to imagine all the things children do during their daily activities, and they will be bound to surprise you with a creative endeavor you never dreamed possible. With their glasses along for the ride, it is of utmost importance to have a frame designed for a child's life.

These are a few of the things you will want to look for in a child's frame:

   1. Sturdy construction:

This means no rimless frames or thin metal frames. They *will* break.

2. Flexible hinges:

    Children will bend glasses in ways contortionists would envy. A spring hinge will help to absorb some of the shock.

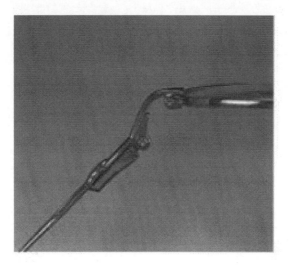

Example of a spring hinge. Notice how it can be bent beyond vertical.

3. Polycarbonate lenses

    This is a little outside the topic of frame selection, but the importance of polycarbonate lenses in children cannot be overstated. Polycarbonate lenses are the most impact-resistant lenses available on the market. For safety reasons, we always want children to be placed in polycarbonate lenses. We will discuss this more in the future chapter on lens options.

Frame selection for the elderly

There is only one thing to keep in mind when fitting the elderly patient: *keep it lightweight!* Elderly patients will have much thinner skin than other patients. They will come back to you with deep red marks where their nose pads make skin contact and ask you to fix it. The only way to prevent this is with proper upfront planning before the problem ever occurs.

1. Choose a lightweight frame, preferably titanium.
2. Stay away from rimless frames. These tend to force the lab to make lenses thicker (and therefore heavier) than otherwise necessary, especially for plus-power prescriptions.
3. Stick with lightweight lens materials such as polycarbonate that we will discuss in the chapter on lens options.

Special considerations for frame selection

The large nose:

What do we do when Groucho Marx comes in for a pair of glasses? How can we help him (and his wife) make his nose look smaller?

1. Use a frame with low, dark, and straight bridges.
2. Use a frame with a light colored rim, or preferably a rimless one.
3. Use a double-bridge frame. This has two bridges, one cutting across the nose at a lower point and thereby shortening the appearance of nose length. However, if a patient has a very short nose, the saddle bridge appears to shorten it too much. For these patients, use a keyhole bridge, which sits higher than normal and gives the illusion of a longer nose.

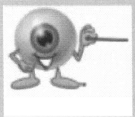 **Focus point:** The Rimless or Semi-rimless Frame: Whenever fitting a rimless or semi-rimless frame, ALWAYS pair it with a polycarbonate lens. CR-39 or high-index lens materials (discussed in a future chapter) will likely crack in such a frame. If a patient refuses polycarbonate, have the patient sign an informed consent form outlining the risks of such a pairing.

The patient with hearing aids:

Fortunately, hearing aids are becoming smaller and are often no larger than the ear canal. However, you will occasionally run across a patient with a large behind-the-ear type of hearing aid. Obviously, the standard-type temple would have a hard time fitting around this type of device. There is no easy way to fit this patient, but there are some things to keep in mind to try to make it easier:

1. The hearing aid temple. There are temples available that are designed with a cut-out for hearing aid devices. These types of temples are becoming more difficult to find and unfortunately are usually paired with some fairly unstylish frames.
2. The cable temple. The cable temple is the thinnest type of temple you can place on a pair of glasses and are the easiest to adjust around a hearing aid as they are extremely thin and pliable.
3. The skull temple. This is a temple that essentially has no bend around the ear. It does not provide the secure fit of the other types of temples; however, the skull temple may be able to fit over the top of a hearing aid.
4. Choose a frame with a little extra length in the temples to allow for adjustment out and away from the hearing aid.

Wide-set eyes:

In order to help draw the eyes into closer proximity, lean toward frames with thick or darker-colored bridges.

Close-set eyes:

Light-colored or clear bridges will appear to widen the distance between the patient's eyes.

Patients with Oxygen Tubing:

Patients who require oxygen tubing and wear glasses are often annoyed by having so much paraphernalia around their face and behind their ears. Many times there is not enough room behind the ears to fit both the oxygen tubes and eyeglass temples. Additionally, there is the cosmetic concern of the appearance of glasses plus the oxygen tubing becoming unsightly clutter on the face. Fortunately for these patients, a recent invention helps. Made by a company called Oxy-view (www.oxyview.com), their Oxyview eyeglasses help solve both these problems.

With Oxy-view glasses, the patient's oxygen tubing is inserted into the end of the temple. The oxygen then travels through a hollow canal within the frame and exits into the patients nose through a small outlet near the nosepads. This means no more visible oxygen tubing anywhere over the ears or around the face. Remember Oxy-view eyeglasses with your next patient who is on constant oxygen therapy. They will thank you for offering them a solution no other optician ever has.

Chapter 3 Test

1. What is the part of the frame that provides support around the ear?
2. List three characteristics a frame should have for fitting someone with high myopia.
3. List three characteristics a frame should have for fitting someone with high hyperopia.
4. What is the single most important consideration when fitting an elderly patient?
5. List two characteristics a frame should have for fitting a child.
6. For a patient with a large, prominent nose, what is the best bridge style?
7. What style frame would you select for a patient with very wide-set eyes?
8. The A measurement plus the bridge size is referred to as what?

CHAPTER 4

Frame and Lens Fitting

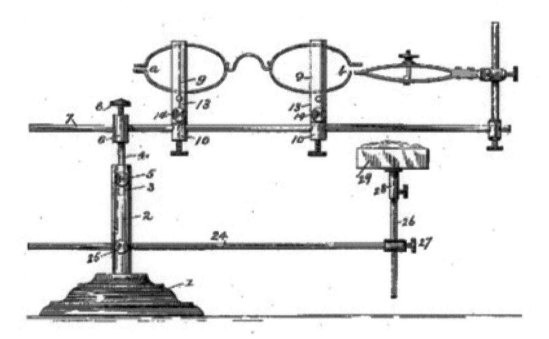

OK, so now you've got this great frame that both the patient and the patient's spouse are happy with. Now you have to turn this frame into a prescription pair of glasses. Doing this is as simple as 1-2-3:

1. Take the patient's PD.
2. Adjust the frame on the patient's face.
3. Measure for bifocal, trifocal, or progressive height.

Measuring Pupillary Distance (PD)

An accurate inter-pupillary distance (PD) measurement when ordering glasses is crucial. This will provide not only clear vision, but also *comfortable* vision. The pupils, you may recall, need to be aligned with the optical center of the glasses. Otherwise, the glasses will induce unwanted *prism*, which will be discussed in detail in the next section, giving the patient headaches and eyestrain.

Typically, you as an optician will not be responsible for actually making the glasses. However, the person who *is* making the glasses is relying heavily on your PD measurement being accurate. This measurement tells him or her where to set the optical centers in the lenses so they properly align with the eyes.

There are several ways to measure the PD of a patient. The easiest and most accurate is with a *pupilometer.*

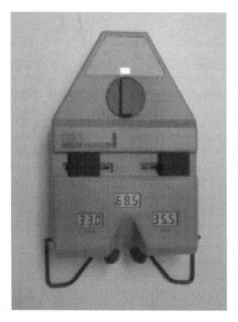
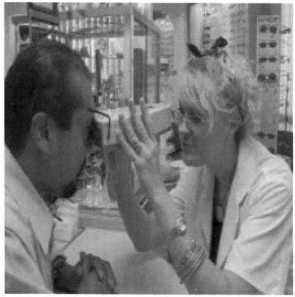

Pupilometer   Use of pupilometer

A pupilometer is an electronic device that helps you measure PD. Of all the methods, it is the most simple to use and provides the most accurate measurement, to 0.5mm. The pitfall of a pupilometer is that it is electronic and susceptible to dead batteries, so it is necessary to know the other methods of measuring PD.

Measuring the distance PD

The patient's distance PD is the distance between the pupils when the patient is in *distance* gaze. This helps the optical lab set the length between the optical centers of the lenses in the distance-vision part of the glasses.

Using the pupilometer

1. Set the dial to measure the patient's distance PD. This will be represented by an infinity symbol (∞).

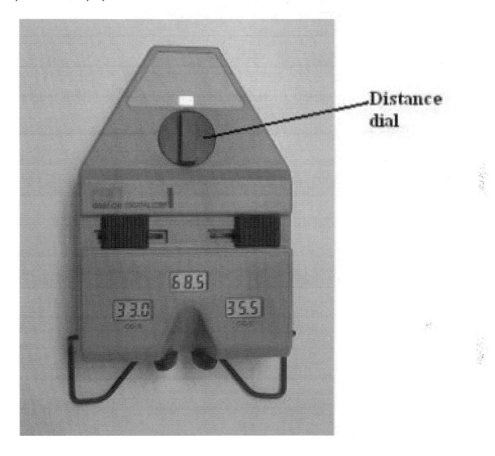

Distance dial

2. Ask the patient to look into the pupilometer as he would a pair of binoculars and to look directly at the small light (usually red or green). The optician looks through the other end.
3. Hold the pupilometer so that your fingers are positioned over each of the measuring slides (there will be one for each eye).

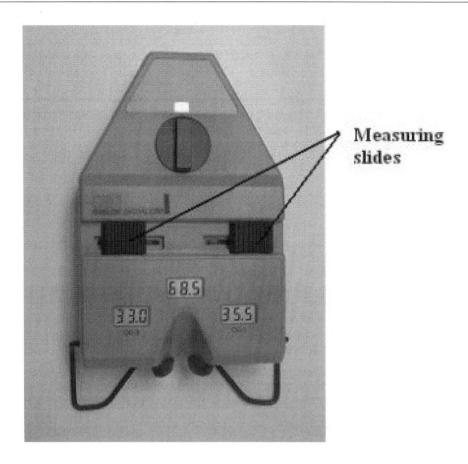

4. Looking through the pupilometer, slide the measuring bars (with the measuring slide you have positioned under your thumbs) until the vertical lines line up with the light reflex on the patient's pupil.

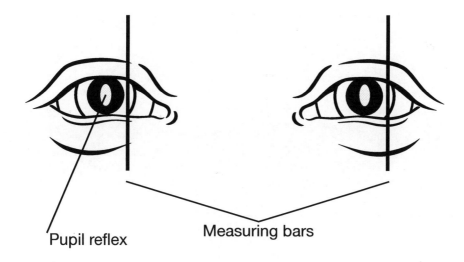

Pupil reflex   Measuring bars

View through the pupilometer before the measuring bars are over the pupil reflex

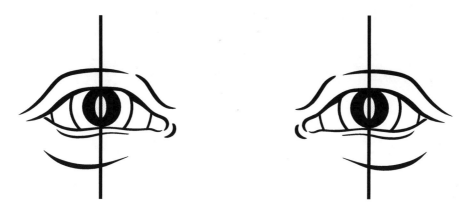

View through the pupilometer after lining up the measuring bars with the pupil reflex

5. Read the digital display for the patient's PD measurement. Most digital pupilometers will give you both the binocular PD (the distance between the pupils) as well as the monocular PD (the distance of each eye from the center of the nose). Monocular PDs, as we will see, are useful when highly accurate PDs are needed, such as for progressive lenses, high index material lenses, or when prescriptions are very strong. An electronic pupilometer is the only way to get a truly accurate monocular PD.

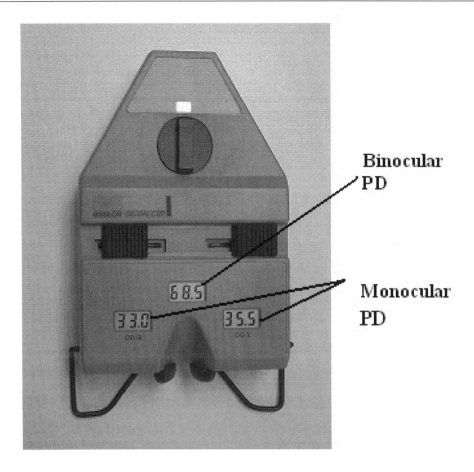

Using the manual method

The manual method has three drawbacks: 1) parallax may skew the measurements slightly; 2) your PD and the patient's PD must be similar; and 3) the patient must have pupils that are the same size. Here are the steps to using this method:

1. Position yourself directly in front of your patient, holding a ruler at about arm's length.
2. Close your right eye (to minimize parallax) and have the patient look at your left eye.
3. Set the "0" mark of the ruler on the right side of the patient's right pupil. Set the ruler on the bridge of the patient's nose for stability.
4. Open your right eye, close your left, and have the patient look at your right eye without moving the ruler.
5. Read the ruler marking at a point that corresponds to the right side of

the patient's left pupil. This is your distance PD. It will likely be in the range of 60-65mm.

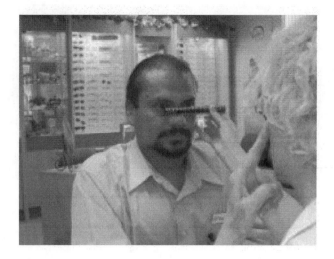

Use of PD rule

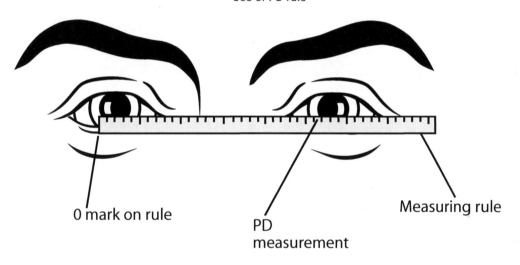

0 mark on rule

PD
measurement

Measuring rule

Your view of the patient's eyes and PD measuring rule

Measuring Near PD

For bifocal wearers or for reading glasses, you also want to measure the patient's near PD so the bifocals can be set at the appropriate location. The near PD will be smaller than the distance PD due to the eyes converging together to fuse an object at a closer distance.

Using the pupilometer

The same technique for using the pupilometer for measuring the near PD is used for the distance PD. The difference is where you set the distance dial. For most reading powers, either for bifocals or reading glasses, the reading distance will be 40cm. However, you must not take this for granted. There are occasional scenarios in which the reading distance will be other then 40 cm.

One of these scenarios is when the reading glasses have been prescribed for use on a computer or for reading music, in which case the working distance would be at arm's length. How will you know when this has been done? Hopefully, the doctor will specify on the prescription that the glasses are "computer glasses" or "music reading glasses." If this has not been done, the only other way is to compare the patient's age with the reading add power. Recall that add powers are very predictably linked to a patient's age. Therefore, if a 70-year-old's reading glasses have an add power of only +1.25 over their distance power, you know these are likely music or computer glasses. You should ask your patient exactly what the glasses will be used for and at what distance. Once you determine the working distance for which the glasses were prescribed, you can simply set the distance dial and take your measurement.

The other scenario in which the working distance will not be 40cm is for cases of bifocal powers greater than +2.50. These strong add powers are typically used in patients with reduced vision from an eye disease in order to help them hold reading material closer to appreciate a sense of magnification. To determine the working distance in these cases, simply take the reciprocal of the add power. For example, if someone is prescribed a +3.00 add, the working distance is calculated by:

Working distance = $1/3 = 0.33$ m or 33cm.

Set the pupilometer distance dial to 33cm and proceed taking your measurement as before.

Using the manual method

You also can measure the patient's near PD using the PD ruler as you did for the distance PD. As a rule of thumb, you should expect your near PD to be approximately 2 to 4 mm smaller than your distance PD. If this is not the case, you may want to re-measure your PDs. To measure the near PD with the PD rule:

1. Sit in front of your patient at the working distance for which their glasses will be used. Recall, you can determine this by either asking the patient at what distance the glasses are intended to be used (40 cm if the add power

is appropriate for the patient's age) or, if the add power is greater than +2.50, using the equation *Working Distance = 1/Add power.*

2. Place your eye in front of the patient's nose at the intented working distance, close your other eye, and ask the patient to look at your open eye.

3. Using your PD rule, place the "0" mark on the left side of the right pupil. Read the measurement from the PD rule that lines up with the left side of the left pupil.

Using the calculation method

It is possible to calculate what the near PD should be in a case in which the working distance is less than 40 cm (add power greater than +2.50). In such a case, getting so close to a patient in order to measure it with the PD rule may be uncomfortable for both you and the patient! To calculate the near PD at these near-working distances for high add powers, use what is called the *three-quarters rule.*

Inset per eye = 0.75 × Add power.

For example, if a patient has a distance PD of 66mm and a bifocal add power of +4.00, the inset per eye = 0.75 × 4.00 = 3mm.

Therefore, *each bifocal* would be inset 3mm compared to the distance PD, making for a total of 6mm less than the distance PD. The near PD would then be 60mm (66mm– 6mm).

It is important to remember that this equation works only in add powers resulting in a working distance less than 40cm (add power greater than +2.50).

Using the lazy-man technique

This technique is used when the add power is in the normal range of +1.00 to +2.50. *Simply subtract 3mm from the distance PD.* For example, using the same patient as in the previous example, the distance PD is 66mm, but the bifocal power is +2.00 instead of +4.00. This time, the near PD is recorded as 63mm (66mm–3mm).

This technique results in a wider near PD than the technique used for higher bifocal powers because of the amount of convergence expected for each strength of bifocal. Remember—from our equation for measuring the working distance of a bifocal or reading glasses—that the working distance is shorter for higher add powers. A shorter working distance means the eyes must converge more; a further working distance means the eyes need to converge less. Therefore, in typical-strength bifocal powers (+1.00 to +2.50), the eyes will converge less than in higher-strength bifocals. Less reduction is required from the patient's distance PD.

Making Adjustments

Adjusting frames will be what you do most as an optician. Despite all your knowledge about optics, for the better part of your day, you will be reduced to being a repairman! However, it will be the most important part of your day as far as patients are concerned. In school, doctors are taught that patients "don't care how much you know until they know how much you care." The same can be said for opticians. If a patient goes home with an uncomfortable pair of glasses, it was because *you* did not care enough to make sure they fit right before they left your office. You can have all the optical knowledge in the world, but one poorly fit pair of glasses will cause that patient to question your skills.

Adjusting frames is 50 percent art and 50 percent engineering. We will now discuss making adjustments to frames using engineering principles. It will take practice to become the artist and to learn how these principles feel in your hands.

A basic goal of all adjustments is to maintain the three-point touch. No, this is not a basketball play; it's how the weight of the glasses is distributed across the face. The two ears and the nose create the three points. There should be equal pressure and weight on all three points to make the most comfortable fit. Keep this in mind as we discuss the various ways in which glasses can be adjusted.

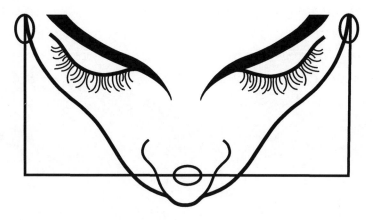

Three-point touch of a properly fitted frame

The Tools

The frame warmer

The frame warmer is an essential tool in making eyeglass adjustments. It heats the frame material, making it more pliable and easier to adjust while reducing the risk of breakage that can occur when adjusting a frame at room temperature. Once the frame cools, the adjustments will remain in place. Remember, however, that some materials hold their adjustments better than others do.

There are two types of frame warmers: one uses a flow of hot air and the other a pan of hot beads. All of these principles will work with either type of warmer. Keep in mind, however, that the warmer that uses the pan of hot beads warms the frame much more quickly, and that the frame may be ready for adjusting after only a few seconds in the pan. Leaving the frame in the pan too long may lead to permanent frame damage, especially on plastic frames.

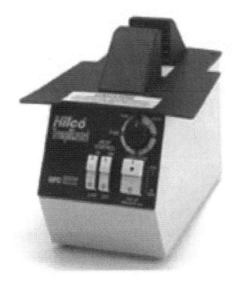
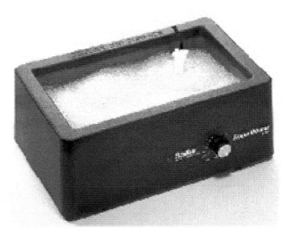

Hot air frame warmer   Pan warmer (filled with hot beads)

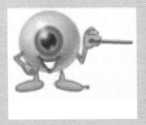
Focus point: Do not leave a frame in a pan warmer for more than a few seconds before trying to adjust the frame. This type of warmer can cause permanent harm to the frame and may even melt the frame after a short time.

The pliers

There are numerous oddly shaped pliers that you will become proficient at using. Once you learn what each tool is for, their odd shapes will begin to make sense to you. We will briefly help you recognize the most common types and later discuss how and why each is used.

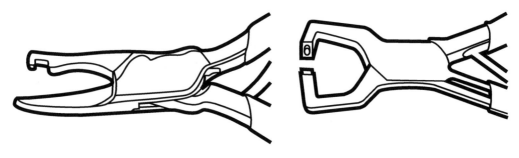

Nosepad pliers   Angling pliers

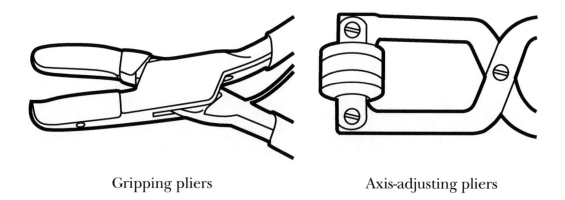

Gripping pliers   Axis-adjusting pliers

1. Nosepad pliers: Adjusts nosepad.
2. Angling pliers: Adjusts temple angle, such as for pantoscopic tilt.
3. Gripping pliers: Holds frame steady for other adjustments without leaving scuff marks.
4. Axis adjusting pliers: Used for making small lens rotation in frame in order to adjust cylinder axis.

The fingers

Your fingers make a wonderful tool for making many of the adjustments necessary on a frame, especially temples. Fingers will not mar the finish on a frame, and you always know exactly how much pressure you are exerting.

The What, Why and How of Making Adjustments

Temple Adjustments

Temples must curve properly around the contour of the ear to be comfortable. A proper curve means it follows the anatomical line of the ear without creating any points of bearing. The inside of the temple should remain in light contact with the skull for its entire length. Any deviation from this and the patient will complain of the frame "pinching" behind the ears.

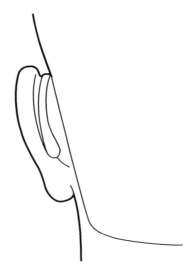

Proper fit of the frame behind the ear follows ear contour

Steps for a proper temple fit:

1. With the frame on the patient, visualize the temple location that must bend around the ear.
2. Heat the temple.
3. Using your finger as a rolling pin, gently mold the temple around your finger until you have formed an approximately 45-degree angle at the location of the desired bend.
4. Place the frame on the patient and examine the temple contour behind the ear.
5. Make an adjustment to the bend location and angle it as necessary to ensure the proper contour. The gripping pliers work well for making fine adjustments to the temple contour. Their padded grips prevent scratching the temple while being used to form the bend around the ear.

Sometimes, you will see a temple on a patient that has a 90-degree bend behind the ear. This is never an appropriate angle, and the patient will be very appreciative if you correct this angle to more closely match the contour of the ear.

Nosepad Adjustments

Nosepads should sit with their entire surface area resting on the nose.

Otherwise, the patient will complain of the glasses "pinching the nose," or the frame will sit too high or too low. The goal is to have the entire surface of the nosepad make equal contact with the nose without an edge making an uncomfortable indentation.

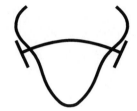

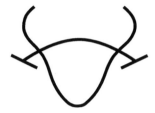

Proper (top) and improper (bottom) nosepad fit

Metal frames will make it easy for you to adjust the nosepad, as most metal frames come with adjustable nosepads. Plastic frames typically have the nosepad molded into the frame, making nosepad adjustment nearly impossible. For this reason, it is essential to check the nosepad fit on a plastic frame before telling the patient, "That frame will be perfect for you!" If the nosepad is not fitting properly, the patient will come back to you the day after picking up these "perfect" glasses, wanting to know why his nose hurts!

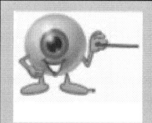

Focal point: Plastic glasses cannot have their nosepads adjusted. Therefore, ensure a proper fit before selecting a given frame for purchase!

This is the basic nosepad anatomy of a metal frame

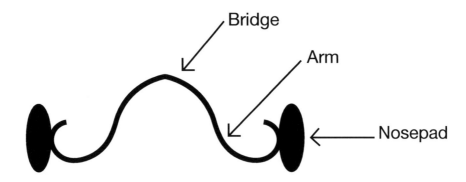

Schematic drawing of a nosepad apparatus

The arm of the nosepad on metal frames will be somewhat malleable. With the use of the nosepad pliers, this arm can be contorted to fit nearly any nose shape or size. This is one of the beauties of metal frames; they make adjustments much easier than plastic frames.

Below are the steps for adjusting nosepads. (Note: not all of these steps will need to be done in every case. The nosepad may already be fitting properly in one regard or another. Keep in mind, however, the effect that adjusting the nosepads may have on the height of the frame on the face and the consequential effect on bifocal heights. How nosepad adjustments affect the fit of the frames in other ways will be discussed later in this chapter.)

1. Grasp the nosepad and arm with nosepad pliers. The groove in the nosepad pliers should fit the nosepad arm like a glove.
2. Adjust the width between the pads to match the width of the nose.

   a. Gently bend the arm outward (toward the lens) to widen the bridge (this also will lower the frame); or
   b. Bend the arm inward to narrow the bridge (this also will raise the frame)

3. Adjust the nosepad landing on the nose. The goal is to have the entire surface of the nosepad in contact with the nose with no edge making an uncomfortable angular contact.

   a. Gently twist the nosepad face inward or outward around the vertical axis if the side pad is digging into the nose.
   b. Gently twist the nosepad face upward or downward if the top or bottom edge of the pad is digging into the nose.

Frame Skew Adjustments

Frame skew is the *levelness* of the frame as it sits on the face. If one side of the frame is either higher, lower, closer to, or further from the face compared to the other side of the frame, a *skew adjustment* must be made. It must be unskewed.

A frame out of skew will cause several problems.

1. It cosmetically will be unacceptable.
2. It likely will cause pressure points on either the nosepads or temples, or both, making the frame uncomfortable.
3. If there is a bifocal, the patient will not use the bifocals simultaneously due to unequal bifocal seg heights.
4. The patient will not be looking through the optical centers of the lenses.

Remembering what needs to be done for each type of skew is easy. Simply remember:

In–In, Out–Out, Up–Up, Down–Down

This refers to what needs to be done to the temple on the side of the skew. For example, what if the right side of the frame sits higher on the face than the left? (This could also be seen as the left side sitting lower.)

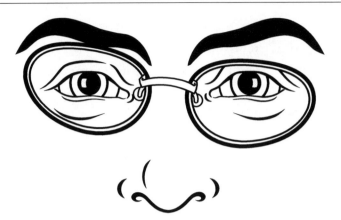

Example of the right side of the frame sitting too high

The right temple needs to be adjusted upward
Or
The left temple needs to be adjusted downward

This admittedly seems counterintuitive. Most new opticians have a hard time grasping the idea that the temple must be adjusted in the same direction as the *skew*. So go ahead and practice this adjustment on a fellow optician. Seeing it in action, and seeing the result if this rule is not followed, will help you remember it for your next patient.

What if the right side of the frame is sitting closer to the face than the left (or, alternatively, if the left side of the frame is further away from the face than the right)?

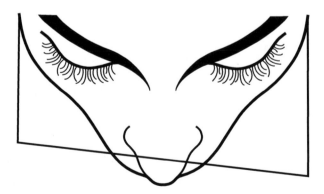

Example of the left side of the frame sitting out too far from the face

The right temple needs to be adjusted inward

Or

The left temple needs to be adjusted outward

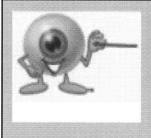

Focus Point: In order to adjust for skew, adjust the temple *on the same side of the skew in the direction of the skew.* Remember: *In–In, Out–Out, Up–Up, Down–Down.* The temple should be bent *upward* on the side the frame is too high, *downward* if it is too low; *in* if it is closer to the face, and *out* if it's further from the face.

Now that we know what needs to be done, how do we do it?

1. Heat the temple hinge in the warmer. This applies mainly to plastic frames; metal frames often do not need to be heated to be adjusted.
2. Using gripping pliers, gently grasp the hinge above the temple to keep it from moving during adjustment. Padded pliers such as these will prevent marring the frame finish during adjustment.
3. Using another set of padded pliers, grasp the temple arm below the hinge and bend it in an appropriate direction using the "in-in, out-out, up-up, down-down" rule.

   a. When adjusting the temple angle up or down, it is best to grasp the hinge parallel to the rim.
   b. When adjusting the angle temple in or out, it is best to grasp the hinge perpendicular to the rim.

   When practicing this, you will understand the mechanical physics behind these grasping techniques.

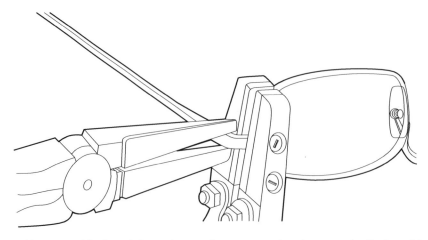

Proper positioning of the tools to make an upward or downward adjustment to the temple

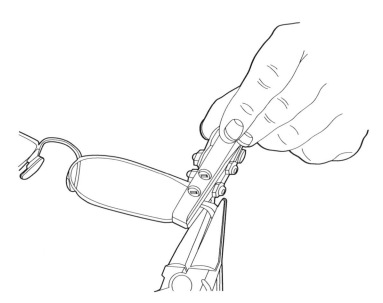

Proper positioning of the tools to make an inward or outward adjustment to the temple

Pantoscopic Tilt Adjustment

When you are going throughout your day, do you find yourself looking directly straight ahead most of the time? Probably not. You are likely looking down slightly most of the time. For example, when walking, you are looking down slightly to see the road 10 feet in front of you. When using your computer, if you have proper ergonomics, you are looking down at the screen approximately 10 degrees. When reading, you are looking down slightly as well. *Pantoscopic tilt* permits the user to look through the optical center of the lens in this slightly downward visual posture. There are times when you *are* looking directly straight ahead or even upward, but the optical center can be at only one location in the lens. Positioning the optical center as if the patient would be looking down slightly most of the day helps the patient use the center most of the time.

Pantoscopic tilt, as defined in "System for Ophthalmic Dispensing" by Clifford Brooks and Irvin Borish, refers to "the angle that the frame front makes with the frontal plane of the face when the lower rims are closer to the face than the upper rims."

Not only does pantoscopic tilt provide the best optical positioning of the lens, it also is the most cosmetically appealing look for the glasses. If the frame front were parallel to the frontal plane of the face, this would be the improper cosmetic result:

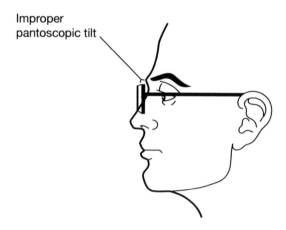

Improper pantoscopic tilt

The pantoscopic tilt should make an angle of approximately 10 degrees on the face. In order to accomplish this, the temples need to be bent slightly at the hinge, with the lower rim bent more toward the face than the upper rim. The following are the steps to achieve proper pantoscopic tilt.

1. Warm the hinge of the frame.
2. With your angling pliers, grasp the hinge and apply pressure, directing the temple downward slightly. Repeat with each temple.
3. Place the frame on the patient's face. Observe the frame fit from the side of the patient and repeat steps 1 and 2 until the desired result is achieved. Your result should look like this:

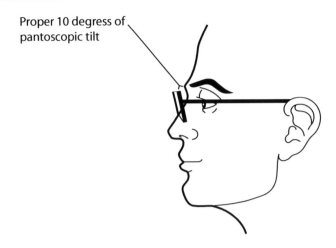

Proper 10 degress of
pantoscopic tilt

This method assumes that the glasses have been measured correctly to begin with. This means the patient's eyes should be looking slightly above the optical centers of the lens when looking straight ahead. If this is not the case, the pantoscopic tilt, although cosmetically more appealing, will not be optically correct. To be correct, the following rule should be applied:

Eyes at optical center	then	No pantoscopic tilt
Eyes above optical center	then	Pantoscopic tilt
Eyes below optical center	then	Negative tilt (not cosmetically practical and will require glasses to be remade)

Vertex Adjustment

The vertex distance of a pair of glasses refers to the distance the lenses sit from the patient's eyes. This is measured with a device called a *distometer*, and typically this distance is about 12–13mm. Ninety percent of the time, you do not need to concern yourself with this measurement. Low or even moderate prescriptions are relatively unaffected by the distance they sit from the eye. However, in cases where a prescription is about 6.00D or greater, you will want to make sure the vertex distance is correct; otherwise the patient will experience a prescription effect different from what is expected.

The optical calculations to arrive at the following conclusion are beyond the scope of this book, but do know this: For any lens prescription, the closer to the eye the lens gets, the more *minus* power the patient will experience. The further away the lens gets from the eyes, the more *plus* power will be experienced. The stronger the prescription, the more this effect is magnified.

Ideally, if the patient's prescription is greater than about 6.00D, your doctor will tell you on the prescription pad the vertex distance of his testing device so you can duplicate that vertex distance in the patient's glasses. But doctors often don't provide this information. So what do you do? In a perfect world, you could call the doctor and ask what the vertex distance should be, but the doctor is not likely to know unless it was documented during the test. The best thing to do is assume a 12–13mm vertex distance. If the patient's current glasses are drastically different from this, you may want to split the difference. In reality, it will be a trial and error process. If a patient with a very high prescription comes back to you with difficulty adapting to a new prescription, but everything checks out with the way the glasses arrived from the lab, you will want to send the patient back to the doctor with a note asking for the vertex distance during testing. This will remind the doctor of both the importance of this measurement and of your excellent optical skills!

The easiest way to adjust for vertex distance is to adjust the temple as previously discussed. If the vertex distance is too short, move the bend in the temple further toward the rear of the temple to allow more room for the frame to sit forward. Similarly, if the vertex distance is too large, move the temple bend forward to snug the frame close to the face.

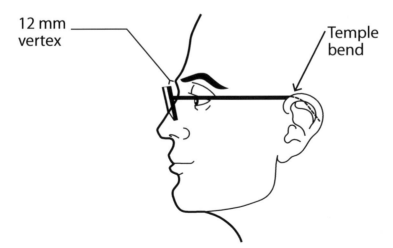

Bifocal height adjustment

One of the most common corrections you will make to a frame is adjusting the bifocal height either up or down. This is necessary for two scenarios: the optician did not have the frame properly adjusted on the face prior to measuring for the bifocal height, or, through normal wear, the frame moved out of place enough to indirectly raise or lower the bifocal line.

There are several things you can do to correct this before resorting to a remake of the lenses.

If the bifocal line is sitting too high (the patient complains that the line gets in the way of distance vision):

1. **Spread the nosepads:** This will drop the frame, and therefore lower the bifocal line.
2. **Increase the pantoscopic tilt:** Due to the angle the lens will make with the face, increasing the pantoscopic tilt will give the illusion of a lower bifocal line.
3. **Decrease the vertex distance:** Similar to increasing pantoscopic tilt, by bringing the lens closer to the face, you will create the illusion of lowering the bifocal line. Be careful, however, not to do this too much for a patient with a high prescription, since changing the vertex distance changes the net power the patient experiences through the lenses.

If the bifocal line is sitting too low (the patient complains of having to push the glasses upward when reading to see through the bifocal):

1. **Bring the nosepads closer together:** This will raise the frame—and the bifocal as a result.
2. **Decrease the pantoscopic tilt:** Creates the illusion of a higher bifocal seg line due to the angle between the lens and the face.
3. **Increase the vertex distance:** By increasing the distance the lens sits from the face, the angle the bifocal seg makes with the eye will give an illusion of a higher bifocal.

Face Form Adjustments:

To be optically correct in most instances, the frame should have what is called *Positive face form.* Face form is the amount of wrap the frame has relative to the contour of the patient's face.

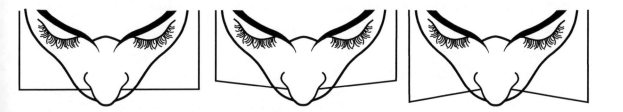

The above illustration shows what various face forms look like when viewing the frame from above the patient's head. Positive face form, the ideal form, occurs when the frame PD ("A" measurement + bridge size) is larger than the patient's PD and is correctly adjusted on the face. In order to adjust the face form:

1. Heat the bridge of the frame (if it is a plastic frame).
2. To add a positive face form: If there is not enough positive face form or negative face form, place your thumbs on the inside part of bridge, hands on the hinges, and gently push your thumbs upward to create the appropriate amount of wrap.
3. To reduce positive face form: Place your thumbs on the outside part of the bridge, with your hands on the hinges, and gently push your thumbs upward to create an appropriate amount of wrap.

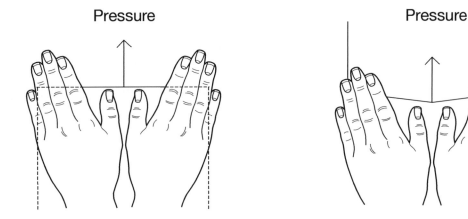

There are some instances when to be optically correct you will want something other than a positive face form. For example, in the rare case in which the patient's PD is larger than the frame PD, a negative face form is required to be optically correct. It is therefore important to steer patients away from such frames during the buying process. If the patient's PD is equal to the frame PD, then to be optically correct there should be no face form on the frame.

In order to be optically correct, follow these general rules:

Patient's PD = Frame PD   *then*   No face form

Patient's PD < Frame PD   *then*   Positive face form

Patient's PD > Frame PD   *then*   Negative face form

In practice, however, try to steer the patient away from any frame that would require either no face form or negative face form to prevent a cosmetically unappealing fit. As a general rule, you can expect most patients' PD to be smaller than the frame PD. Occasionally, you may run across one of the exceptions, so try to be aware of the frame PD when you are measuring the patient's PD so you know what type of face form is required and can select the best possible frame.

Prescription axis adjustment

The cylinder axis in a pair of glasses can be adjusted slightly after the lens is ground and placed into the frame. If the lens has been ground by the lab more than a few degrees off axis, the lens must be remade. However, if it is only a few degrees or less off axis it may be able to be savaged with the use of the axis-adjusting pliers.

To do this, grasp the lens that is off axis with the axis-adjusting pliers so that the plier pads grasp on each side of the lens. With gentle pressure, rotate the lens within the frame in the needed direction (clockwise or counterclockwise) in order to match the axis with the needed prescription. After each small rotational movement, check the axis in the lensometer to confirm that you are rotating in the correct orientation and to see how much further you have left to go. This technique typically only works if you need to adjust the axis by less than three to four degrees.

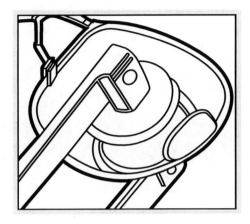

Rotating the lens to adjust the cylinder axis

Measuring for Bifocals, Trifocals, and Progressives

The accurate measurement of multifocal lenses requires properly adjusting the frame on the face, which is why we discussed adjustments first. If you wait to adjust the frame on the patient after you measure the bifocal height, there is a good chance your adjustment will place the bifocal higher or lower than you intended for it to be. *Therefore, it is essential that you completely adjust the frame on the patient before proceeding to measure bifocal, trifocal, or progressive seg heights.*

Bifocals

It is essential to measure the bifocal to sit at the proper height. A bifocal that is set too low will force a patient to push the glasses upward to read.

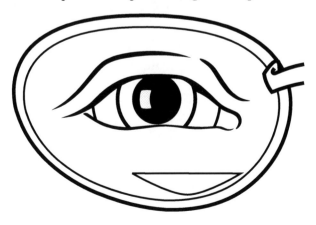

Bifocal set too low

A bifocal set too high will force a person to slide it down to the tip of the nose in order to see over it for the distance portion of the lenses.

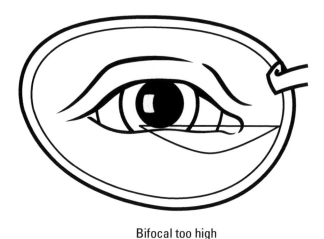

Bifocal too high

A bifocal measured correctly should allow the patient to look through the distance portion of the lenses without noticing the bifocal line, and to gaze downward only slightly for the reading power. The upper line of the bifocal (called the seg) must sit at precisely the proper location, the lower eyelid.

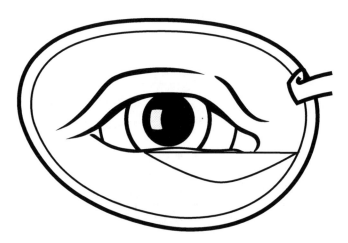

Correct placement of bifocal line

To make this seg height measurement, follow these steps:

1. Make sure the frame is properly adjusted on the patient.
2. Have the patient look straight ahead over your shoulder.

3. With a wet-erase Sharpie pen, place a line on the lens location that corresponds to the lower eyelid. (Most frames in your dispensary will have a plastic lens for marking already inserted into the frame. If not, use a piece of clear tape to wrap around the frame on which to make your mark).

4. Measure from the upper edge of the *lowest part* of the lower rim to your marked line. The lowest part of the lower rim may not necessarily be in line with where the bifocal will be, but this is the location the lab uses to set the seg height. Add 0.5 mm to this measurement, since the actual cut lens will sit slightly in the rim groove. This is your bifocal (seg) height measurement. There will be a place to record this measurement on your order form.

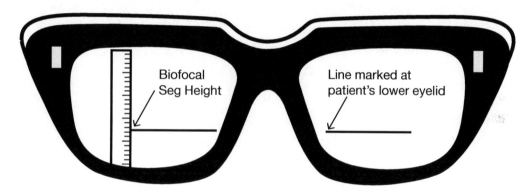

Remember these steps, because they will remain the same for measuring for trifocals and progressives except for the location to mark.

Trifocals

It is just as essential to have trifocals set at the proper height. Again, the top line of the trifocal is called the "seg," and the distance from the bottom rim to the seg is called the "seg height." If we were to set a trifocal seg height at the same spot we set a bifocal seg height, the reading portion of the trifocal would be too low to be useable without pushing up the frames every time the person wanted to read.

In order to position a trifocal accurately, follow the same steps you did for a bifocal, but place your marked line at the position of the *lower pupil margin*.

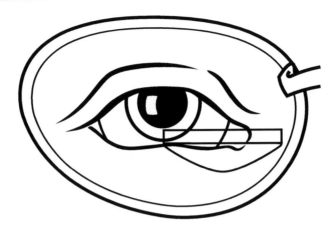

Correct placement of trifocal

This will accomplish several things:

1. The patient will still have a direct straight-ahead view through the distance portion of the lens without the trifocal lines getting in the way.
2. The patient will have the intermediate portion available with only a slight downward gaze.
3. The reading portion will not be set uncomfortably low for reading.

Keep in mind that typically a patient will look down only slightly for most intermediate tasks (imagine looking at a speedometer or at your computer screen). Now imagine how far down you typically look when you're reading (such as a book on your lap or a newspaper on a table). You will notice that you look down much further when performing near-reading tasks than when you look at intermediate objects. This is the premise behind the design of the trifocal. Distance vision is straight ahead, intermediate vision requires a slight downward gaze, and near tasks require further downward gaze.

It is important, however, to keep in mind what patients have become accustomed to in their seg heights. Be sure to ask your patients if they are happy with the seg position in the glasses they currently have. Some patients may have in their current glasses a seg height that looks completely too high or too low, yet they are happy with its location. In a case such as this, *do not try to be the hero; keep the seg height at the same location as in their current glasses unless they are having problems!*

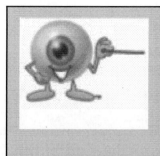 **Focus point:** Always properly fit and adjust the selected frame to the patient before making any lens measurements such as bifocal height! Not doing so will lead to disastrous consequences when the prescribed glasses are ultimately dispensed and necessary frame adjustments throw off the bifocal height or optical centers.

Progressives

Progressives, as you will recall, do not have a line defining where the distance power ends and the intermediate or reading powers begin. Progressive lens manufacturers, in their infinite wisdom, decided you needed a third way to measure a seg height. Progressives do not have an actual seg line, but we still do need a way to measure at what height the intermediate and reading powers should begin. Out of convenience, the term *seg height* is applied to progressives as well even though there is no true seg line.

Progressive lens manufactures design their lenses to have the seg height measured at the center of the pupil. All of the other steps remain the same as in bifocal and trifocal height measurements, but instead of marking the lens for measurement at the lower lid (bifocal), or the lower pupil margin (trifocal), you will mark the lens at the center of the pupil. As before, the seg height is from the lower rim of the frame to this mark, plus 0.5mm for the frame groove.

In addition to seg height, be sure to also:

1. Specify monocular PDs. Accurate monocular PDs will ensure the progressive corridor is well positioned over each eye.
2. Ensure that the frame has 10 degrees of pantoscopic tilt and is properly adjusted prior to making measurements. Pastient satisfaction with progressive lenses is most dependent upon well-made measurements to ensure proper optical accuracy.

Chapter 4 test

1. Before making any lens measurements, such as bifocal height, what must be done first?
2. In order for the glasses to be made with the optical centers appropriately spaced in front of the patient's eyes, you must be certain to make an accurate measurement of what?
3. A pupilometer is used for what purpose?
4. The near PD should be measured at what distance?

    a. 40 cm

    b. 33cm

    c. The proposed working distance

5. In order for a bifocal to be positioned correctly, it should be lined up with what anatomical structure?
6. The seg height of a progressive addition lens is measured from where?
7. What is the basic goal of all frame adjustments?
8. If the left lens is closer to the patient's face than the right lens, what two adjustments can you make to fix the problem?
9. For a proper fit, how many degrees of pantoscopic tilt should be present?
10. What are three adjustments that can be made to a frame to address the concern of the bifocal line getting in the way of distance vision?
11. What is the primary source of patient satisfaction with progressive lenses?

CHAPTER 5

Lens Options

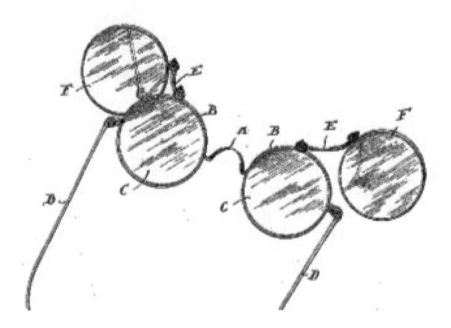

LENS options are the additional features of a lens that make it lighter, stronger, more cosmetically appealing, or more functional. These lens options will usually be an additional cost to the patient, so it is important to understand the benefits of each option to best meet the patient's wants and needs.

Standard plastic lenses, also called CR-39, have been the most commonly used lenses for many years. Compared to its predecessor, glass, CR-39 is lighter-weight, more impact-resistant, and tints better. Patients like it because it is less expensive than some of the newer lenses. But even if CR-39 is your workhorse lens, there are many benefits to the newer materials that may make them a preferred choice for certain patients.

High Index

The higher the power prescribed in a pair of glasses, the thicker the lens will tend to be. This is where high-index lens materials become useful. These materials refract light more efficiently than conventional plastic lenses. Recall that the higher the index of refraction, the greater ability it has at bending light. This means less lens material is needed to correct the same amount of prescription. So what are the advantages of this?

Thinner lenses. Because of the greater ability to bend light, lenses made of high-index materials are thinner than the same prescription made from conventional plastic material.

Lighter lenses. Since the lenses are thinner, this will often reduce the overall weight of the lenses, so they are more comfortable to wear.

There are many high-index materials, which are typically denoted by their "index of refraction." Any material with an index of refraction higher than that of conventional plastic is referred to as "high index" or sometimes "mid-index." High-index lenses are available ranging from indexes of 1.53 to 1.8. For comparison, a standard plastic lens has an index of 1.49. The higher the index number, the thinner the lens will be. All other things being equal, a lens made from a 1.66 index material will be thinner than a lens made from a 1.56 material. Also, generally speaking, the higher the index, the higher the cost.

Let's look at a few examples to help clarify how this index value is used.

A basic, no-frills plastic lens has an index of refraction of 1.49. Whether or not this will be thinner or thicker than another lens of the same prescription depends on how this index of refraction compares with the index of the other lens material. Another lens, a high-index lens, has an index of 1.6. This lens will therefore be thinner than the standard plastic lens. A third lens, also made of a high index material, has an index of 1.8. This third lens will be thinner than the 1.6 lens and *much* thinner than the plastic lens.

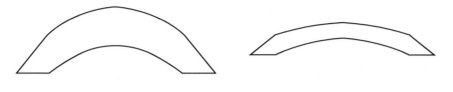

Plastic + 5.00 lens   High-index + 5.00 lens

High-index materials will thin a lens

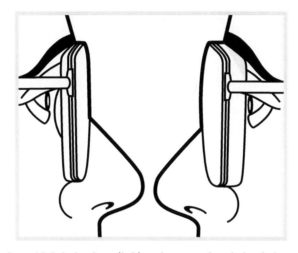

Comparing a high-index lens (left) and conventional plastic lens (right)

Two other important aspects of high-index material are specific gravity and Abbe value. Specific gravity is a measure of the material's weight. Exactly how this is measured is beyond the scope of this book, but know that the higher the specific gravity, the heavier the lens per ounce. Therefore, a lens with a high index of refraction may help to make a lens thin, but to have the ultimate thin *and* lightweight lens, you must also select a material with low specific gravity. Therefore, making a small increase in index of refraction from, say, 1.57 to 1.58, will make a minimal improvement in lens thinness. If there is a large increase in specific gravity in the 1.58 compared to the 1.57, it may not be worth having the mildly thinner lens due to the increased weight. Let us look at a few examples of this. Refer to the "Lens Material Choices" chart on the following page.

1. A standard plastic (CR-39) lens has a specific gravity of 1.32. Polycarbonate has a specific gravity of 1.20. Therefore, ounce for ounce, poly will be lighter weight than plastic.

2. A high-index 1.66 lens has a specific gravity of 1.35. Polycarbonate, with its index of 1.59, has a specific gravity of 1.20. So although the 1.60 high-index lens will be thinner than a polycarbonate lens, the polycarbonate lens may actually be lighter weight due to its lower specific gravity.

Specific Gravity   Weight

1.0

1.2

1.4

1.6

2.0

As specific gravity goes up, weight goes up.

The other element that is useful to look at in high-index lenses is the Abbe value, a measure of how much the wearer will observe *chromatic aberrations.* These appear as distortions, oftentimes colored, that are seen if the patient looks away from the optical center of the lens. High-index lenses will create this effect more often than standard plastic or glass lenses. Just to make things difficult to remember, the *higher* the Abbe value, the *fewer* distortions will be present

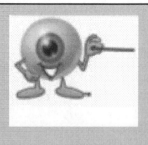

Focus point: In order to minimize the aberrations on higher-index lenses induced by low Abbe values, be certain to specify monocular PDs on your order to minimize the patient from looking outside the optical center of the lens. Adding an antireflective coating to high index lenses can help minimize this feature of high index lenses even further.

Standard plastic lenses have an Abbe value of 58. Polycarbonate has an Abbe value of 31. Therefore, patients wearing poly are more likely to notice aberrations than those patients wearing plastic lenses. Keep in mind, however, that not everybody notices the aberrations. If someone is having a hard time adapting to his new poly lenses and his prior lenses were made of plastic, these aberrations may be to blame. Despite this drawback, polycarbonate lenses will still likely be your number one choice of lens for all of the previously discussed reasons.

Abbe Value   Abberations

30

40

50

60

As Abbe value increases, aberrations decrease.

Lens Material Choices

Material	Index of Ref	Specific Gravity	Abbe
Glass	1.52	2.54	58
Plastic	1.49	1.32	58
Polycarbonate	1.59	1.20	31
Trivex®	1.53	1.11	44
High Index 1.56	1.56	1.42	39
High Index 1.58	1.58	1.42	37
High index 1.60	1.60	1.34	37
High Index 1.66	1.66	1.35	33
High Index 1.71	1.71	1.41	36
High Index 1.74	1.74	1.46	34

High-index lenses provide an option to meet a wide variety of patient needs. For patients who need higher-power lenses, you can provide a lens considerably thinner than a lens made of standard plastic. For children and people exposed to the danger of flying objects, polycarbonate high-index lenses provide a level of safety not found in any other lens. For elderly patients whose skin is thin and easily irritated by excessive weight, you can provide a lens that is lighter weight than any they have ever had. You can be these patients' hero!

To maximize high index sales, be sure your office has demos! Showing how much thinner a high-index lens is than a standard plastic lens will nearly always sell the high-index lens. Many optical labs will offer to make you a demonstration kit of high-index lenses; all you have to do is call to ask. Labs know it's good for sales. It becomes a win-win for both the lab and the retailer.

Polycarbonate

Polycarbonate is a type of high-index lens. It is thin and lightweight like other high-index lenses, but it has some extra features that make it a very appealing option. Polycarbonate ("poly") was the first high-index lens introduced and is still the most widely used. Compared to other high-index materials that are currently available up to an index of 1.8, polycarbonate has a modest index of 1.59. But poly shines for other reasons. It is the standard for safety glasses and for children's glasses due to its impact resistance. Poly can withstand impact forces much greater than any other lens material without shattering. In addition, polycarbonate provides excellent inherent UV protection without having to pay extra for a UV coat application to the lens. It has low *specific gravity*, which means, ounce for ounce, that poly is lighter than other lens materials. Polycarbonate should be the only lens material used in rimless or semi-rimless frames, any other material will likely crack in such a frame. Finally, poly's impact resistance allows a laboratory to ground it thinner than any other material, to 1.0mm. So although poly may not have the highest index, these advantages place it on a level playing field with the other higher index lenses.

With all these good points, you are probably wondering whether there are any disadvantages to poly. Polycarbonate is a very soft material and therefore is more prone to scratches. For this reason, most labs will automatically apply a scratch coating to poly lenses. Additionally, due to this soft property, polycarbonate lenses are more prone to aberrations, possibly adding to some unusual visual symptoms. These aberrations, measured by a material's *Abbe value*, will be discussed in more detail in the next section. Polycarbonate is also more difficult to tint, especially in dark shades.

Despite the drawbacks, choosing polycarbonate as a lens option is often easy to justify. It is lightweight, thin, has UV protection as an inherent property, is very safe, and typically has a scratch coat automatically applied. Even with all these benefits, polycarbonate lenses are often quite economical. Polycarbonate is certain to be one of your most used lens materials

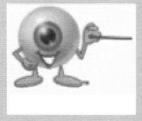

Focus point: For safety reasons, polycarbonate needs to be your lens of choice for all children under the age of eighteen. You and your prescribing doctor can be held legally liable if your young patient does not receive polycarbonate lenses and receives an eye injury while wearing some other material that shattered. Be certain that if a parent ever refuses polycarbonate for his or her child for any reason, that you document this in the chart and have the parent or legal guardian sign a waiver underlining the risks of not having the child in polycarbonate lenses.

Trivex

A new competitor to Polycarbonate has recently hit the market. The material is known by its trade name Trivex®. Like polycarbonate, Trivex is considered a mid-index material and has inherent UV protection. It's very low specific gravity, however, can make it as lightweight as many high index materials for a lower cost.

Trivex has many benefits lending to its recent popularity. The impact resistance of Trivex is comparable to Polycarbonate. However, using this in place of polycarbonate for children is not recommended at this time. Polycarbonate is still considered the standard of care for children in most ophthalmic circles. We have not been able to find a court case where the selection of Trivex instead of polycarbonate in safety glasses was claimed to have been the cause of an ocular injury. Therefore, there is no precedent to predict how the court system would view your choice of lens material. It is always preferable to stay with the standard of care rather than risk setting a precedent in court. Be safe and always use polycarbonate for your under-18 year of age patient and in safety glasses. Its impact resistance, however, is an excellent selling point for those patients who do not fall within the above mentioned polycarbonate-required groups but still want a high safety profile.

A second benefit of Trivex is its light weight. Although having an index of refraction more similar to standard plastic CR-39 than its' mid-index sibling, Polycarbonate, the specific gravity of Trivex is significantly lower than polycarbonate and even lower than any high-index material (see Lens Material Choices table). This lower specific gravity in mid range prescriptions, such as +/-3.00D to +/-6.00D could create a lighter weight lens than by using a more expensive higher index material.

A third benefit of Trivex is its relatively high abbe value. Compared to polycarbonate and other high index materials with a lower abbe value, Trivex's higher abbe will create fewer chromatic aberrations. Therefore, consider this lens for someone you deem to be a "poly non-adapt" patient. The term "poly non-adapt" is used for a patient in polycarbonate, usually for the first time, who has vague symptoms of not seeing well despite all troubleshooting efforts yielding no benefit. Many times changing such a patient into a higher abbe value material will solve the complaint.

Aspheric Lenses

An aspheric lens, in the technical sense, is any lens that incorporates *various* curvatures as opposed to a uniform curve throughout the lens. "A" as a prefix means "not," and "spheric" means symmetrically curved. Therefore, an aspheric lens is a lens that has a different curvature in the center of the lens than it does in the periphery. In the optical world, aspheric lenses are used to gradually flatten the thick part of lenses in order to make them cosmetically thinner and subsequently lighter weight. You will often combine the aspheric option with the high-index option to create an extremely thin and lightweight pair of glasses.

There are three major benefits of aspheric lenses.

1) **Weight and thickness**. An aspheric lens can dramatically reduce the thickness of high-power lenses by flattening the area of a lens that is otherwise the thickest. This would be the center part of a plus-power lens or the edge of a minus-power lens. By having less lens material, the lens will also be much lighter weight.

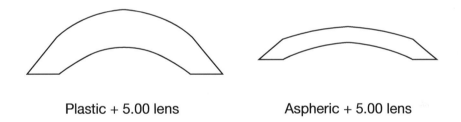

Plastic + 5.00 lens   Aspheric + 5.00 lens

An aspheric lens will be thinner than a regular lens

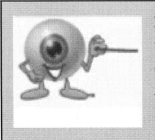 **Focus point:** Due to the flat nature of an aspheric lens, unacceptable reflections may be present without the use of an antireflective coating. *Always* be sure to include an AR coat with all of your aspheric lens orders.

2) **Better vision**. An aspheric lens can reduce the off-axis aberrations experienced by patients when they look through the edges of

non-aspheric lenses. On a non-aspheric lens, the further away from the center the patient looks, the more distortions appear. Aspheric lenses correct for this with their continually modified curvature.

3) **Cosmetically more attractive.** An aspheric lens will reduce the magnified appearance of the wearer's eyes, making for a more cosmetically appealing pair of glasses. In plus-power lenses, the thicker the lenses, the more magnified the wearer's eyes will be. Ordering the lens to be aspheric, and therefore thinner, will help your patient feel less self-conscious of this effect while wearing the glasses.

The key to promoting an aspheric lens is in demonstrations. Your office likely has a demonstration model that compares lenses of equal power, one aspheric and one not. If your office does not have such a demo, ask that your lab make you one. It will be the single best demonstration device you can use.

When discussing aspheric lenses, or any lens option to a patient, try to avoid technospeak and stick with the benefits. For example, aspheric lenses do not "utilize a gradual alteration of the curvature in order to minimize lens thickness and maximize non-abberated vision," but rather will "provide you with an incredibly thin and lightweight lens which will also maximize your vision and make you look great!"

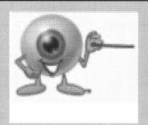 **Focus point:** Combining an aspheric lens with a high-index material will give you the ultimate in a thin and lightweight lens.

Since aspheric lenses are generally flatter on the back surface than non-aspheric lenses, the patient may complain of what is often called "lash-crash": the patient's eyelashes rub against the lens with every blink. Try to select a lens that maximizes the *vertex distance* (the distance between the eyes and the back surface of the lens).

With all the benefits to the patient of aspheric lenses also comes added responsibility by the optician to ensure a proper fit. As with a high-performance car, you must take a little added care to ensure you give patients the full benefit of their investment. Remember the following keys when ordering an aspheric lens.

1. Take monocular PDs. This allows you to center lenses over patients' eyes more accurately than a binocular PD.

2. Select a frame in which about 10 degrees of pantoscopic tilt can be achieved.

3. Specify to the lab the vertical location of the optical center. To do this, first mark on the lens the location of the pupil in a straight-ahead gaze. Then, measure from the lower rim of the frame to this mark. Now, subtract 1mm for every 2 degrees of pantoscopic tilt. For a typical 10-degree tilt, subtract 5mm. This is sometimes referred to as the "Rule of Tilt."

Another, sometimes easier, way to measure this vertical location is called the Head Tilt method. Have patients hold their head so that the lenses and floor are perpendicular. Have the patient look straight ahead, and mark the pupil location. This mark now gives you the desired vertical height of the optical center without having to estimate the pantoscopic tilt.

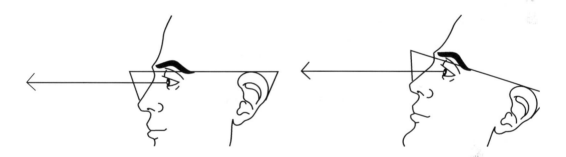

Rule of tilt method. The patient is in normal gaze and the location of the pupil is marked on lens. The optical center is recorded as being this height minus 1mm per 2 degrees of tilt.

Head tilt method. The patient tilts his head until frame is perpendicular to the floor and looks straight ahead. The pupil location is marked. This is your optical center height.

Scratch-Resistant Coatings

No eyeglass lens material is scratch-proof. However, a lens that is treated with a scratch coat does become more resistant to scratching. Most types of plastic lenses, including high-index and polycarbonate, have scratch-resistant coatings automatically placed on them during manufacturing due to their softer nature.

Most scratch coatings are inexpensive and will come with a one-year warranty against normal scratching, making it a good investment.

In general, glass lenses will scratch less easily than plastic lenses, and plastic lenses will scratch less easily than high-index lenses. You may occasionally run across a patient wearing glass lenses that feel like they weigh a ton; the patient is willing to sacrifice weight in order to have the extra scratch resistance glass lenses provide. Scratch coats typically come with a one-year warranty, but don't be surprised if the patient insists on staying with glass lenses.

You should discuss scratch protection with *all* patients, especially those who work in dusty, dirty environments.

Ultraviolet Treatment

A lens treatment that is beneficial, but invisible to the naked eye, is ultraviolet (UV) protection. Similar to the way that sunblock prevents the sun's rays from damaging the body in the form of a sunburn, UV protection shields the eyes from the same light rays that are thought to cause such things as macular degeneration, cataracts, and skin cancers around the eyelids.

Ultraviolet treatment is inexpensive, quick to apply to most lenses, and does not change their appearance. Keep in mind that UV protection is inherent in most high-index lenses, such as polycarbonate. UV protection, in the form of a UV treatment or a lens that has the protection inherent, should be discussed with everyone. UV protection for the eyes cannot be overemphasized.

Antireflective Coatings

To improve both vision and appearance, an antireflective coating (AR coat) is applied. AR coatings consist of several layers of metal oxides applied to both sides of the lens. Each layer progrevely blocks reflections from the lens. This benefits the patient in several ways. The patient will see a reduction in nighttime glare, a great safety benefit when driving at night. The coating also will help cut the glare created from a computer screen or an overhead reading lamp.

Additionally, an antireflective coating reduces reflections on the lenses themselves when viewed by another person, creating a cosmetically more natural-looking lens on the face. With an antireflective coating, lenses appear non-existent in photos and are unnoticeable to people looking at the wearer. All of these benefits are even greater with higher prescriptions.

Combining an antireflective coating with high-index lenses and polycarbonate is not just a good idea. It is required for the best optical outcome. An AR coat can minimize the aberrations the patient experiences in low Abbe-value materials such as poly and other high-index materials. Additionally, high-index lenses have light transmission values only in the high 80-percent to low 90-percent range due to loss from reflections. This can give the patient reduced night vision and even occasional daytime eyestrain. Adding an AR coat brings light transmission back to nearly 100 percent in these lenses by reducing reflected light. Always pair high-index and polycarbonate lenses with an antireflective coating for this reason.

As discussed previously, aspheric lenses, due to their flat curvature, will create more reflections than non-aspheric lenses. Aspheric lenses should *always* be paired with an antireflective coating. This is such an important pairing, that some labs automatically pair aspheric lenses with an AR coat.

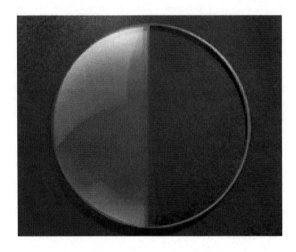

A lens without antireflective coating (left) and with (right)

With sunglass lenses, an AR coat applied to the back surface of the lens helps reduce the reflections of light that enter from behind the wearer and bounce off the tinted surface into the wearer's eyes. The darker the sun tint, the more noticeable these back surface reflections will be. An AR-coated sun lens is much more visually comfortable than an uncoated sunglass. You should recommend a back-surface AR coat on all sunglasses.

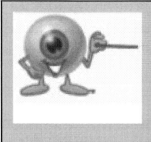

Focuspoint: All high-index lenses, including polycarbonate, have low Abbe values compared to traditional plastic lenses. They also transmit less light. Patients using these high-index or polycarbonate lenses, therefore, should always have an antireflective coat applied to their lenses. This will reduce the aberrations induced by the low Abbe values and increase light transmission through the lens.

Polarization

A polarizer is a lens that filters the "visual noise" reflected from horizontal surfaces such as water or streets. You have probably seen the annoying glare from your horizontal dashboard reflected in your windshield. All of these glares are reduced with the use of polarized sunglasses.

How does this work? Think of glare as a water balloon hitting a flat surface. The water splashes in all directions! It's the same with sunrays hitting a flat surface. They create reflected light in all directions: horizontally, vertically, diagonally, and every other way. This chaotic pattern of light rays creates the visual disability associated with glare. Polarized treatment to sunglasses filters this glare so that only light rays approaching the lenses in one particular orientation are allowed to pass though to the eye. Similar to watching a dog try to carry a long bone through a door that is only slightly ajar, polarized lenses block all light rays that do not have just the right orientation for the polarization.

Fishermen greatly appreciate polarized sunglasses. The polarization eliminates the glare from the surface of the water and allows the user to see schools of fish underneath.

Photochromatics

Photochromic lenses change from light to dark as you go from indoors to outside, then lighten again as you return indoors. This makes photochromatics a great choice for professions that require continually walking between indoors and out, such as real estate or construction. Without photochromatics, these patients would constantly have to switch between their clear glasses and sunglasses.

The darkening mechanism in photochromatic lenses is a chemical called *silver halide*. When exposed to UV light, the molecules are excited into a state of darkening. The more UV light exposure, the darker the lenses become.

Photochromic lenses do not darken very well inside a car because most windshields block out UV rays. So for people who want driving sunglasses, it is best to recommend a separate pair that is permanently tinted. Additionally, the performance of photochromatics is temperature dependent. They will darken better on bright, cool days than on hot, sunny days.

First-generation photochromics were strictly glass lenses, but today you can choose from plastic, polycarbonate, or other high-index materials. Lenses are available in nearly every lens design and prescription. New features include advanced technology that allows more rapid darkening when you go outside (and a more rapid return to clear when you go inside), and 100 percent UV protection. In the newer formulas, the coating darkens evenly regardless of lens prescription or thickness; in previous generations, glasses did not darken well on the thicker parts of the lens.

Tints

In contrast to the changeable photochromics, another option in colored lenses is a permanent tint. Tints are available in almost any color desired. Lighter tints are used often as a fashion accent, while darker tints allow the wearer to use the lenses as sunglasses when paired with a UV coat.

A tint can be solid—in which the entire lens is the same color—or gradient, a gradual fade from dark to light, usually fading from the top down. Tints are relatively inexpensive and often can be bleached out of the lenses if patients change their mind about the color. Keep in mind that *a tint alone does not provide UV protection*. To truly make a pair of sunglasses, you must combine the tint (for comfort) with a UV coat (for protection).

Mirror Coatings

These coatings are bold in color and highly reflective. Choices include every color of the rainbow as well as silver, gold, and copper. Mirror coatings are excellent at reducing light transmission and are therefore ideal sunglasses for people frequently outdoors who want the maximum in light blockage. A common application of a mirror coating is a *flash mirror* coat. This is a thinner mirror coat for those who do not want an obvious mirror finish to their sunglasses.

The color chosen for the mirror coat is 50 percent cosmetic and 50 percent science. Patients often have a particular mirror color in mind for cosmetic reasons, but you can offer them some science to help with their decision. For sport enthusiasts, orange, brown, yellow, and amber will help to improve contrast. Gray, green, and plum are good for glare reduction. Gray reduces light transmission evenly across the color spectrum, so it is a good choice for the patient who does not want any perceived color change to their viewing environment.

Adding a mirror coating can reduce light transmission through the lenses more than the darkest tint alone. This is due to the high amount of light being reflected from its surface. As an added benefit, the light rays that mirror coatings reflect is disproportionately in the form of harmful UV and infrared light. As with any sunglasses, be sure to add a *backside* antireflective coating. The darker the lens, the more reflections the patient will experience.

Progressives

Progressives, as you may recall, are a newer type of multifocal lens that do not have the lines inherent in bifocals and trifocals. This is possible through rapid changes in the base curve of the lens. Progressives have two inherent benefits over their previous generation multifocals:

1. Without lines, many patients perceive them as cosmetically more appealing.
2. They have a point on the lens corresponding to every distance in space. Technically, they could be called *infinite-focal* lenses. Many people refer to progressives as a no-line trifocal, but this would be an insult to the progressive lens. The benefit a trifocal lens has over a bifocal is that it fills in the gap between distance and reading, such as computer work. The jump from a trifocal to a progressive is similar. Even a trifocal technically creates an unmet focal distance need between distance and intermediate, and again between intermediate and reading distances. Progressives fill in these gaps.

As with most good things in life, there are some trade-offs. Progressives have two main ones.

1. Peripheral distortions. In order to get the optics to blend without a line, the rapid base curve changes create peripheral distortions. The higher the add power, the more dramatic these peripheral distortions become, especially in the reading area.

2. Because of these peripheral distortions, the field of view is narrower than with bifocals or trifocals.

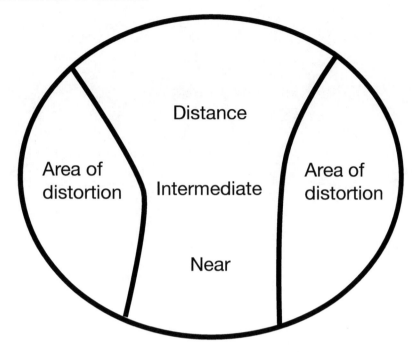

A schematic diagram of a typical progressive lens.

Not all progressives are alike. There are hundreds of different brands, and each brand has a slightly different arrangement of optics and distortions. It helps to think of progressive designs as falling on one of two ends of a spectrum, either hard or soft. Hard progressives maximize reading area but have more peripheral distortion, and soft designs have minimal distortions but typically less reading area.

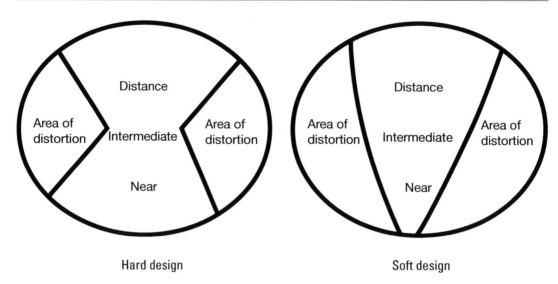

Hard design   Soft design

Additionally, as discussed previously, there are "short corridor" progressives. These shorten the area between the distance and reading powers to help them fit better into small frames. This type of progressive has areas of distortion more similar to the hard design.

It is important to educate patients of this distortion prior to ordering the lenses; otherwise they *will* be back with complaints. The better you educate, the better the patients adapt to the lenses. The following are some keys to help with patient education on progressives.

- Never say "distortions." It is better to say "curvature changes." This makes it sound more intentional (which technically it is) than unintentional.

- Explain that the patient will need to turn their head for a clear view instead of looking through the edge of the lens when viewing peripherial objects..

- Fully educate patients on the visual advantages of the progressive lens over the bifocal or trifocal. This will help them be more motivated to adapt.

- Call patients a few days after they pick up their glasses. This will give you another chance to answer questions about issues they may have forgotten, such as the peripheral distortions (oops, power changes) or about having to turn their head towards what they are viewing.

Digital (freeform)

There has a rapid rise in the number of digital, or "freeform", lenses manufactured in the last few years. There has been an equal amount of confusion on the part of patients and opticians alike regarding what this really means. We aim to give you a basic understanding to the world of digital lenses and explain what makes them unique.

What makes a digitally manufactured lens different from a standard one?

A standard lens starts as a semi-finished premolded lens with a standard base curve on the front surface. The manufacturing lab will then generate the Rx on the back surface of the lens without altering the foundation of the design already molded on the front curve.

A digitally surfaced lens, in contrast, uses software which takes into account prescription, pantoscopic tilt, vertex distance, frame fitting position, and sometimes even eye movement patterns, to create a "customized" design for each particular patient. In theory, this will provide greater definition in all viewing angles. The outcome, as a result, is unique for the given patient's prescription. Contrary to common belief, it is not the lens itself, but rather the process by which the surface of the lens is manufactured.

No two lens manufactures use the exact same software to create their digital lenses. Therefore, each optical boutique cannot possibly be proficient at fitting every type of digital lens available, especially digital progressives, as they all will have slightly different fitting requirements. Most offices will chose one or two digital lens manufactures in order to become proficient in their digital lens fits.

Due to the lens design being based on many parameters, including the frame shape, the prescription in a free form lens is referred to as a "compensated Rx". Conventional lenses are designed to maintain best clarity when viewing straight ahead. Digital technology attempts to provide that same clarity in all viewing angles. This optimized Rx is called the "compensated Rx", which is the prescription you will see when analyzing it in the lensometer, not necessarily the same as that which was prescribed, especially true with progressives.

The lens manufacturer will provide you with a card along with the digital lenses with the "compensated Rx" you will find analyzing the lenses in the lensometer. Digital lenses are accurate to 0.01 diopters, which is why you may see "compensated Rxs" not written in 0.25 steps like doctors prescribe.

Possible pitfalls

Just because a lens uses the word "digitally processed", does not automatically mean a patient will like it more than a non-digital lens. The benefits are dependent upon:

1. Abilities of the processing lab.
2. Software designing the digital lens.
3. Accuracy of the data provided by the fitting optician.

Because there is so much more required accuracy involved on the part of the lab and the fitting optician, there is also less room for error. Any error the optician provides the lab, such as an incorrect PD or seg height, will become much more magnified than in a standard lens design. Standard lens designs can absorb small errors more easily without patients perceiving the problem.

For a patient who has been a long time successful lens wearer without complaints, it may be hard to justify changing them into a digital design. However, if a patient has historically been unable to adapt, especially to progressive lenses, a digitally designed lens may provide a beneficial second chance.

Top 5 take away things to know about digital "freeform" lenses

1. Placing the word "digital" on the lens does not automatically make the patient happier than with what the patient is already wearing.
2. Success with digital lenses require the perfect balance of 1) A good software design, 2) a good measure of all required parameters by the optician, and 3) a good fit of the frame to insure it fits exactly as it was when the measurements were taken.
3. Get to know how to fit a couple brands really well. Unlike standard lenses, you will never be proficient at fitting all of them since each brand has slightly different fitting requirements.
4. The potential benefits of freeform lenses is tremendous. However, it is hard to justify using a digital lens, especially progressive, in lieu of a patient's current progressive if they are already happy. For previous PAL non-adapts, it might make sense to give a digital PAL a try.
5. The "compensated prescription", the prescription as read through the lensometer, may be noticeably different from the prescribed Rx values. Do not be surprised by this. Most freeform lens manufactures will send you a "Compensated Rx" verification card along with the lenses.

Don't be afraid to jump in and get your feet wet with this technology if you have not already, this is the future of lens technology so the more you gain experience with them now the sooner you will learn how to use it to the patient's best advantage.

Chapter 5 test

1. Children should always be placed in what lens material?
2. What are two benefits of antireflective coatings?
3. Why should an AR coat be applied to polycarbonate lenses?
4. Which lens will be thinner: a lens with an index of 1.59 or one with an index of 1.66?
5. Combining a high-index material with what other lens property will result in the ultimate in a thin and lightweight lens?
6. Why should you always add an antireflective coating to an aspheric lens?
7. When could a high-index lens actually weigh more than a lower-index lens?
8. What can be done to a lens to reduce the chromatic aberrations caused by a high-index material, such as polycarbonate?
9. What are two potential problems associated with aspheric lenses?
10. If a patient wants sunglasses made, what two lens options at a minimum *must* be included?
11. What is the benefit of adding an antireflective coat to sunglasses?
12. What are two advantages and two disadvantages of progressive lenses?

CHAPTER 6

Contact Lenses

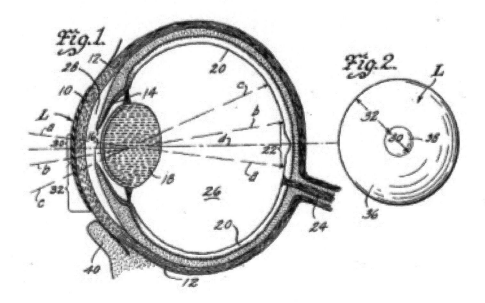

CONTACT lenses are one of the most fun areas in the eye care field …
for the patient. For you, the optician, it can be a nightmare of paperwork
and training on the application and removal of lenses. This chapter will
help you understand how to train someone on the use of contact lenses, the care
and handling of the lenses, and how to find specifics about contact lenses when
needing to place an order.

First, though, let's give you some basics about contact lenses. There are
generally two types of contact lenses, hard and soft. Hard lenses, also known as
rigid gas permeable, have been around the longest, dating back to about the 1940s.
Hard lenses have become the exception rather than the rule in recent times for a
variety of reasons, but they will always have their place in certain cases, as we will
discuss.

The benefit of hard lenses is two-fold. One, they can last several years or longer with proper care. You may see many patients who have been wearing the same hard lens for a decade! Two, they can correct many eye conditions that soft ones simply cannot, such as high amounts of astigmatism or keratoconus (a misshapen cornea). In such cases, the rigidity of hard lenses is necessary mask the irregular shape of the front corneal surface, thereby providing a higher level of optical quality.

The pitfall to hard lenses is the initial adaptation to comfort. A hard lens will not be as comfortable as a soft lens initially, but a majority of patients will get accustomed to it. In this age of instant gratification, not all patients are willing to wait a week to a month for the lens to begin to feel comfortable, however.

The benefit of soft lenses is also two-fold. The first is that soft lenses, unlike hard ones, are disposable in most cases. Several brands are even designed to be thrown away daily. This feature is useful for patients who have a tendency to lose their lenses or tend to have tears that deposit protein on the lenses, causing them to become cloudy over time. The pitfall to soft lenses is their limited use in irregular corneas such as in high amounts of astigmatism. Soft lenses will not give the optical quality needed in such cases that hard lenses provide through their rigidity.

Comparison of Hard vs. Soft Contact Lenses

	Pros	Cons
Hard	Best optical quality	Initial discomfort
	Lasts sometimes decades	Lacks disposability
Soft	Disposable	Lacks optical quality for some Rxs
	Good initial comfort	Limited range of powers

Soft lenses come in a variety of options:

1. Yearly
2. The 2-week to 1-month disposable (the most commonly used)
3. The daily disposable (quickly becoming the lens of choice for many doctors)

And a couple of lens materials:

1. The conventional material (silicon), which cannot be slept in
2. Silicon hydrogel, which may be slept in for one week to a month at a time with a doctor's approval.

Here are a few of the most common contact lens-related terms you may hear and will want to know:

1. Soft contact lens: A flexible contact lens. Usually disposable.
2. Hard (rigid gas permeable, or RGP): A rigid contact lens. Not disposable.
3. Spherical: A contact lens that does not correct astigmatism.
4. Toric: A contact lens that corrects astigmatism.
5. Multifocal / Bifocal: A contact lens that corrects distance and near vision simultaneously.
6. Disposable: A type of contact lens that is thrown away anywhere from on a daily basis to monthly.
7. Conventional: A soft contact lens that is not thrown away for an entire year.
8. Colored / Opaque: A contact lens designed to change a person's eye color.

Contact lens cleaning solutions have come a long way in the last ten years. There was a time not long ago when cleaning contact lenses was a three- or four-step process. One solution was used to clean the lens, one disinfected the lens, one removed protein buildup, and one rinsed the lens before reapplication to the eye. Most of the modern solutions are *multipurpose solutions* that are able to do all of these steps in one bottle. We will discuss the proper cleaning of contact lenses shortly.

Training a patient on the application and removal of lenses will likely become a common practice in your work place. We will now discuss how to do this and look like a pro! There are some major differences between applying and removing hard and soft lenses. We will discuss the hard lenses first.

Application and removal of hard contact lenses

To apply a hard lens to the patient's eye:

1. Wash your hands well and be sure to rinse all soap residues away. Have a lint-free cloth available for the patient to dry her eyes when they begin to water, which they will when the patient is learning to insert a rigid contact lens for the first time.

2. Place the lens on the tip of your index finger, concave side up. Use your right index finger if you are right-handed, your left if you are left-handed.

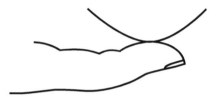

3. Place the index finger of your other hand on the upper eyelid close to the eyelash margin and raise the eyelid. With the middle finger of the hand with the contact lens, pull the lower eyelid downward. *Having good control over the eyelids is essential.*

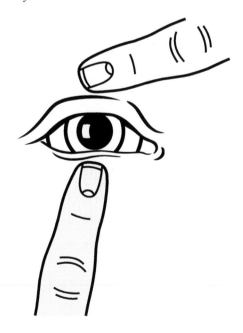

4. Instruct the patient to look straight ahead, and with the index finger holding the contact lens, make gentle contact with the lens onto the cornea. The lens should easily remain in place on the cornea as you pull your finger away.

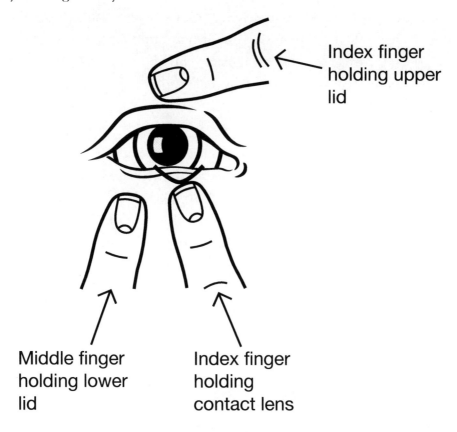

Index finger holding upper lid

Middle finger holding lower lid

Index finger holding contact lens

6. Release control of the lids *slowly!* A sudden release of the lids, which causes them to clamp down over the contact lens too quickly before the lens has a chance to settle, can turn the lens into a flying projectile! Watching pro athletes on their hands and knees looking for a contact lens is funny; being the one having to do it, however, is not!

7. You have done it! Now get going on the other eye

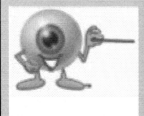

Focus point: Manufacturers of hard lenses place a small black dot on the lens of the right eye. This is to help you and the patient know which lens is for which eye.

To have the patient apply a hard lens to his or her own eye:

Simply repeat the same steps, but obviously using the patient's fingers and a mirror for the patient to look into. Patients use the same fingers when applying the lens themselves as you use when you are doing it for them. When selecting the index finger hand to hold the contact lens for insertion, select the index finger on the hand opposite from the eye the lens is being inserted into. This makes the lid support a little more efficient.

Always instruct the patient to have a clean working environment and to insert lenses over a solid countertop, not a sink, so that the lens does not get lost down the drain! Additionally, it is helpful to have a colored washcloth or towel on the counter under the patient's head to make finding the lens easier should it fall. There are few things more difficult than finding a clear lens on a white countertop!

To remove a hard lens from a patient's eye:

A *greenie* is a device designed for the removal of hard contact lenses.

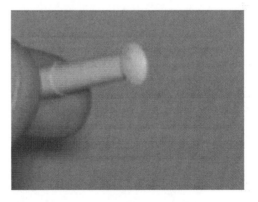

"Greenie"

It is a soft, rubber, handheld plunger (typically green, hence the name) that when placed on the contact lens will suction to it and remove it from the eye. Extra caution must be made with this device, however, since **severe harm can be caused to an eye if the bare eyeball is plunged with the greenie**. For this reason, rarely do we allow patients to use a greenie on themselves to remove a contact lens. However, they can be useful for us to remove a contact lens when other methods fail.

To use a greenie to remove a contact lens:

1. Visually locate the contact lens on the eye. **DO NOT TAKE THE PATIENT'S WORD THAT A CONTACT LENS IS ON THE EYE.**
2. Slightly moisten the suction-cup end of the greenie with saline and place it directly on the center of the contact lens at a perpendicular angle.

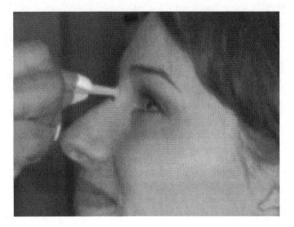

3. Pull the greenie away. The contact lens should be firmly suctioned on the end of the greenie and removed easily from the eye. You may hear a small "*pop*" break in suction as it is removed from eye.
4. **Gently** remove the lens from the greenie

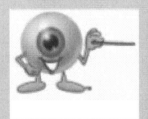 **Focus point:** Before removing a contact lens with a greenie, make certain you visually locate the contact lens on the eye. Do not use a greenie on an eye that you simply assume has a contact lens on it. Serious damage can occur to the eye if you use a greenie on an eye without a contact lens or simply fail to plunge the lens and instead plunge the eyeball.

To remove a hard contact lens without *a greenie:*

There are a couple of methods. Practice with each method and find the one that is easiest for you.

The Pinch-off Method:

1. Wash your hands and rinse off all soap residue.
2. Sit the patient over a table to catch the lens if it falls.
3. Have the patient look straight ahead.
4. Place one index finger on the upper eyelid margin and one on the lower eyelid margin, directly adjacent to the upper and lower contact lens edges.
5. With gentle inward pressure, bring your two fingers toward one another slightly.

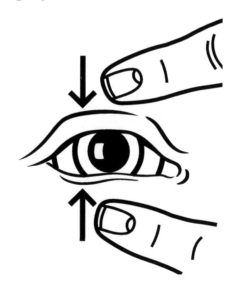

6. The lens should pop out as the eyelids catch under the upper and lower edges of the contact lens.

The Tug-and-Blink Method

1. Wash your hands and rinse off all soap residue.
2. Have the patient look straight ahead with eyes wide open. The patient must be able to open his eyes wider than the diameter of

the contact lens for this method to work. For older individuals with floppy eyelids, this likely will not be the best method.

3. Tighten the eyelids by gently pulling outward on the outer corner of the eyelids. Have the patient blink with her hand under her cheek to catch the lens as it falls out.

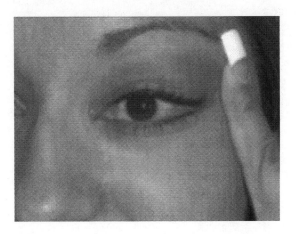

To teach a patient to remove a hard lens from his or her own eye.

Never allow a patient to go home with a greenie. A well-intentioned patient who tries to remove a contact lens with a greenie when the lens is not actually in the eye can do serious and permanent damage.

Both the Pinch-off Method and the Tug-and-Blink Method will work by the patient on themselves. The Tug-and-Blink Method is probably the most widely used, but find the one that works best for you and your patients and use it as your first line of training. Keep in mind that not all methods work for everyone, and some patients create their own very creative methods. As long as it is not a method that will cause harm to the eye, or to anyone else standing nearby, let the creative juices flow! However, I do recommend becoming proficient at these two methods before you start trying to get too creative with other methods.

To recenter a hard contact lens:

Oftentimes, a patient will come into the office with a hard lens that has become decentered off the cornea and onto the white sclera, and ask you for help to get it recentered. It is a good idea to include recentering training with all of your new contact lens patients. This will prevent the proverbial five o'clock Friday afternoon patient knocking on your door for help.

To recenter the lens:

1. Have the patient look in a direction away from the side of the eye the lens is on.
2. With your index finger, gently support the outer edge of the lens.
3. Have the patient slowly return to looking straight ahead.
4. As the patient looks straight ahead, your finger will act as a roadblock keeping the lens stationary. The patient's eyeball will slide under the lens, and the lens will become recentered.

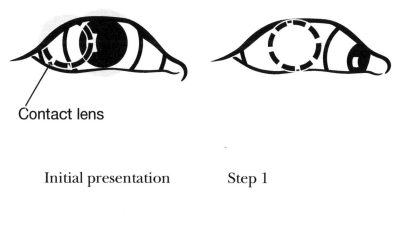

Contact lens

Initial presentation   Step 1

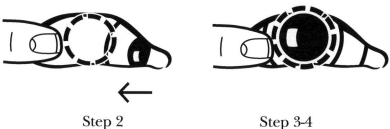

Step 2   Step 3-4

Steps in recentering hard lens

Application and removal of soft contact lenses

Soft contact lenses are more easily damaged than the rigid variety of lens. First-time wearers must be properly trained in their application and removal to avoid costly tears that can occur in the soft lenses.

Apply soft lenses in much the same fashion as hard lenses. However, soft lenses tend to be much larger, so it is even more important to have good control over the eyelids to ensure they are out of the way for lens insertion. *Eyelids and eyelashes getting in the way are the biggest obstacle to successful lens insertion.*

Application of a soft contact lens:

1. Wash your hands and have a clean work environment.
2. Place the contact lens concave side up on the index finger opposite the eye it will be inserted into.
3. Ensure the lens is right side up.

    a. Unlike hard contact lenses, soft lenses by their very nature are capable of becoming inverted. An inverted lens will not cause any harm to the eye, but it will make the lens much more irritating and may slightly decrease the patient's vision.

    b. To tell if a lens is right side up:

        1. Place the lens on the tip of a finger and look at it in profile.
        2. If the lens looks bowl shaped, smooth and even along the edges, the lens is likely right side up. Otherwise, flip the lens over and inspect again.

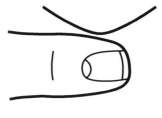

Correct

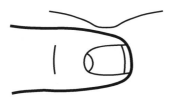

Incorrect

Proper orientation of soft lens prior to insertion

4. Apply the lens as described for hard contact lenses. Soft lenses, unlike hard lenses, will have a tendency to center themselves once applied. Therefore, if the patient is hesitant with your finger (or even his or her own finger) coming directly at the eye, you may place the lens on the white part of the eye and then move the eye toward the lens to achieve centration. Additionally, if the soft lens and finger are too wet, the lens may stick to the finger and not transfer to the eye. If you find this happening, simply dry your finger with a lint-free cloth and try again.

5. Instruct the patient not to blink immediately. A hard blink too soon after insertion will likely fold the lens and cause it to fall out of the eye. The lens must settle for a few seconds before the lids close. After a few seconds, you may instruct the patient to *gently* close his or her eyelids and *gently* massage the closed eyelids to remove any air bubbles that may be under the lens.

Removal of soft contact lenses

Some opticians and patients have an easier time removing hard lenses, others soft. The basic mechanics of removing a soft lens are simple, but do take some practice to master. Like riding a bike, once you learn how, it becomes an easy task.

To teach a patient to remove a soft contact lens from an eye:

1. Wash your hands and have a clean work environment. Make sure to have your cleaning supplies and a mirror nearby.

2. Look upward or to the side, exposing a large area of the sclera (the white part of your eye).

3. With your middle fingers, support the upper and lower eyelids, making sure to get eyelashes out of the way.

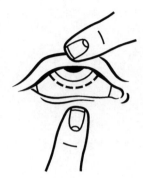

4. With your index finger, slide the contact lens onto the exposed white part of the eye.

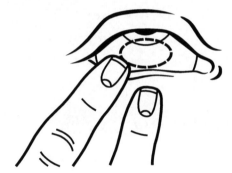

5. Without releasing your index finger from the lens (otherwise the lens will just recenter itself again), gently pinch the contact lens with your index finger and thumb and remove from the eye.

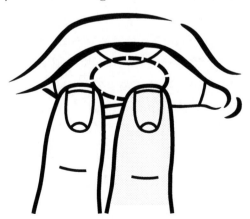

6. Proceed immediately with cleaning and storing.

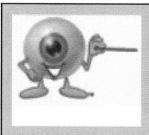

Focus point: Never remove the contact lens from the eye by pinching it directly off the cornea. The cornea, the clear part of the eye, is very susceptible to damage. The sclera, the white part of the eye, is much tougher and can tolerate your finger pinches much more readily.

To remove a lens from a patient's eye yourself, follow these similar steps:

1. Have the patient look upward or to the side.
2. Support the patient's upper and lower eyelids.
3. Slide the lens to the white part of the eye with your index finger.
4. Pinch off.
5. Clean and store.

Contact lens cleaning, disinfection, and storage

Fortunately, for all of our patients as well as for us, contact lens care and cleaning have come a long way in recent years in terms of convenience and effectiveness. This is largely because of the introduction of soft disposable contact lenses. By throwing away your contacts every two weeks to a month, they never have a chance to build up the protein that the older cleaning systems had. There are even contact lenses available now that you throw away after each use, eliminating the need for cleaning solutions altogether.

Another advance that has greatly improved the convenience of cleaning solutions is the introduction of *multipurpose solutions*. These combine cleaning and disinfection into one step. You can be thankful that you came along when you did into the field of eye care. Although we have more options than ever before in the type of contact lenses we fit for a patient, the care of these lenses no longer requires a chemistry degree!

There are four things we must do to a contact lens (and therefore the solution must do) at the end of the day to ensure it is properly cleaned and disinfected for the next day's wear:

1. Clean: Cleaning a contact lens removes the debris that builds up on a

lens during normal daily wear. The mucus, dust, and any other particles on the lens must be cleaned off before the next step, disinfection, can be accomplished. Therefore, a solution must be capable of breaking through these foreign substances on a lens without damaging the lens itself.

2. Disinfect: Disinfecting a lens means removing harmful bacteria.

3. Enzymatically clean: A patient's tears will eventually deposit protein on a contact lens, and enzymes can clean it. Protein film will make the lens less comfortable, less oxygen-permeable, and reduce the patient's vision, so having a lens free of protein buildup is important. As lenses become more disposable, this step is becoming less vital.

4. Rinse: Prior to reinserting the lens the following day, the lens must be rinsed free of the solution it was soaked in overnight to remove anything that may have settled on the lens. (The exception is with hard contacts. You would lose some of the conditioning effect the solution performed on the lens.)

As you can see, it is a mighty tall order to ask one solution to do all four of these things. However, fortunately, these solutions are available and today are the standard of care. In years past, all four of these steps were separate solutions, so you can imagine how complex cleaning was and how lucky we are today. There are still times when using multiple solutions is the preferred method, and we will discuss when these times are. But these multipurpose solutions will be your solution of choice 95 percent of the time.

Proper care, cleaning, and handling of hard contact lenses

Now that we have the contact lens out of the eye, what do we do with it?

Boston makes a wonderful multipurpose hard contact lens solution called, aptly, Boston Simplicity. This solution will clean, disinfect, store, and rinse hard contact lenses; it will also *condition* the lens to make it more comfortable upon application to the eye. All hard lens care systems, whether a multipurpose solution or a multistep process, have a component that conditions the lens. Hard contact lenses are, by definition, hard. The eye typically does not like hard things put into it. The conditioning properties of the solution, therefore, aim at providing a cushioning-type effect when the lens is placed in the eye.

So what is the process of cleaning a hard lens with Boston Simplicity (or any hard lens one-step solution)?

1. Be sure to have clean hands and a clean work environment. Have your solution and storage case nearby. Always start with the same lens so the patient develops a routine and will not forget which lens she is working with.

2. Clean: Place a few drops of the solution on the contact lens and rub gently in the palm of your hand with your index finger. Repeat this process for both sides of the lens. The mechanical action of your finger combined with the solution will dislodge debris from the lens.

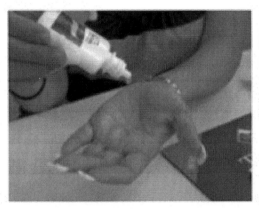   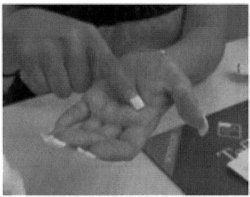

Placing cleaner on lens   Rubbing lens with cleaner

3. Rinse the lens with multipurpose solution. For hard lenses, it is OK for patients to rinse with tap water, and patients will admit they do this regularly to save money by not using as much solution. However, never recommend this to a new patient. Tap water impurities will not absorb into a hard lens like it will a soft lens, and, as you will learn, if you give patients an inch, they will take a mile. If you allow them to cut this corner, they may be tempted to cut others. So for safety's sake, train them to rinse their lenses with the multipurpose solution. A better option than tap water, and more economical than using the multipurpose solution, would be to use saline solution, which is basically just sterile water. It is relatively cheap and can be found at any grocery store, so it is a good alternative for patients who balk at the expense of the multipurpose solution.

4. Disinfect: Fill half the storage case with the multipurpose solution and place the lens in the case. Then fill the remainder of the case with the

multipurpose solution. Store the lenses for at least four hours, but preferably overnight. As the lenses soak in the solution, the antimicrobial properties kill any germs on the lens and condition the lens so insertion is more comfortable the next morning.

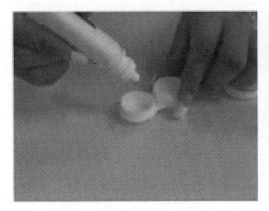 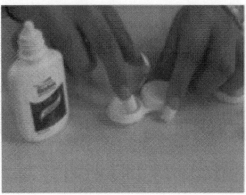

Preparing case for lens   Inserting lens into case for storage

5. Repeat with the other eye.
6. In the morning, remove the lenses and place them in the eyes. No rinsing is necessary or even recommended at this stage. It would only remove the conditioning and make the lens less comfortable.
7. Occasionally, a doctor will notice unacceptable amounts of protein deposits on the lens. If this is the case, he may prescribe an *enzymatic cleaner* for the patient. These solutions typically involve just placing one drop in the storage case along with the multipurpose solution for overnight soaking.
8. After the lens is inserted, the case should be rinsed with hot water and allowed to air-dry.

Boston Original™ (or Advanced) is a multisolution system that is also very popular for cleaning hard contact lenses. Your office may use this instead of the Boston Simplicity™. If this is the case, these are the steps for the Boston Original™ or Advanced system:

1. Be sure to have clean hands and a clean work environment. Have your solution and storage case nearby. Always start with the same lens so the patient develops a routine and will not forget which lens she is working with.

2. Clean: Place a few drops of the RED CAP cleaner on the contact lens and rub it gently into the palm of your hand with your index finger. Repeat this process for both sides of the lens. The mechanical action of your finger, combined with the solution, will dislodge debris from the lens. The red cap on this bottle is a sign that you *never* want this solution on the lens when it is placed in the eye.

3. Rinse the lens with saline solution.

4. Disinfect: Fill half the storage case with disinfection/conditioning solution and place the lens in the case. Fill the remainder of the case with the same solution. Store the lenses for at least four hours, but preferably overnight. As the lenses soak in the solution, the antimicrobial properties of the solution will kill any germs that may be on the lens as well as condition the lens to make insertion more comfortable the next morning.

5. Repeat with other eye.

6. In the morning, remove the lenses and place them in the eyes. No rinsing is necessary or even recommended at this stage. It would only remove the conditioning and make the lens less comfortable.

7. Enzymatic cleaners may be added to the system for additional protein removal.

8. After the lens is inserted, the case should be rinsed with hot water and allowed to air-dry.

You will notice that with the multi-solution system, there are two extra bottles, the cleaner and the saline. The cleaner in the Boston Original™ system is a little more effective than in the Boston Simplicity™.

There are many hard contact lens cleaning systems available to the patient at any grocery store. Boston, however, is the most doctor-recommended and used brand. All brands, however, use the same basic cleaning regimen.

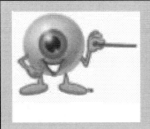 **Focus point:** In the event of any lens discoloration or eye irritation with contact lenses, tell patients to contact their eye care professional immediately.

Proper care, cleaning and handling of soft contact lenses

Just like with Boston Simplicity™ for hard lenses, the most common soft-lens cleaners are also one-bottle multipurpose systems. Optifree™, Renu™, and Complete™ are the most commonly used multipurpose soft-lens systems on the market, and your office is likely to use one of these. Soft lenses are easily torn, so women with long fingernails must be careful during the cleaning process.

To clean a soft contact lens:

1. Be sure to have clean hands and a clean work environment. Have your solution and storage case nearby. Always start with the same lens so the patient develops a routine and won't forget which lens she is working with.
2. Clean: Place a few drops of the multipurpose solution on the contact lens and rub gently in the palm of your hand with your index finger. Repeat this process for both sides of the lens. The mechanical action of your finger combined with the solution will dislodge debris from the lens.
3. Rinse the lens with multipurpose solution, *never with tap water*. It has many impurities that can become absorbed into a soft lens. A patient may use saline solution as a cheaper alternative.
4. Disinfect: Fill the storage case halfway with the multipurpose solution and place the lens in the case. Fill the remainder of case with multipurpose solution. Store the lenses for at least four hours, but preferably overnight. As the lenses soak, the antimicrobial properties of the solution kill any germs that may be on the lens.
5. Repeat with the other eye.
6. In the morning, remove the lenses and place them in eye. No rinsing is necessary at this stage.
7. Rinse the case with hot water and allow it to air-dry.
8. As with hard contact lenses, there are enzymatic cleaners for soft lenses the eye doctor may recommend. The most common of these is Supraclens. As with the hard-lens enzymatic cleaner, use only one drop in the case as the lenses are soaking overnight. Most disposable lenses do not need this step, since the lenses are disposed of before protein has a

chance to build up. However, some patients are in the same soft lens for the entire year and will definitely need an enzyme protein remover for their lenses.

Are these steps starting to sound familiar? They ought to. Whether cleaning hard or soft lenses, the same actions must occur: cleaning and disinfection. With the disposability of soft lenses, enzymatic cleaners for protein removal are rarely necessary.

In certain cases, a doctor may recommend a *hydrogen peroxide* lens care system. These systems are better at dealing with certain bacteria and viruses than the multipurpose solutions. In individuals with conditions that compromise their body's own immune system, such as HIV or diabetes, these hydrogen peroxide systems may be the safest choice. AOSept™ is the most commonly used. The regimens for using these systems vary by brand and are considerably more complex than the multipurpose solutions. You should read the instructions provided with such systems or have your team leader, manager, or doctor show you how to use it.

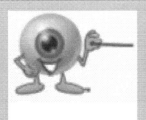 **Focus point:** When not using a multipurpose solution, it is important to remember that cleaners do not disinfect, disinfectants do not clean, and that saline solution (a solution for rinsing) does not clean or disinfect.

Storage of lenses between uses

Most contact lens wearers may go a week or more between wears. Many use their contacts only during certain times of the year, such as for social occasions or sports. So what must be done with the contact lenses during these long periods of storage?

Storage for up to one week: Lenses may be stored for one week. The lenses should be recleaned with fresh solution no more than forty-eight hours prior to lens reinsertion.

Storage for up to one month: Lenses must be recleaned with fresh solution at the end of every week of storage, when the antibacterial action of the solution begins to diminish. As with one-week storage, the lenses also must be recleaned no more than forty-eight hours prior to reinsertion. Read the product insert if you are using a solution not cited in this book.

Storage for more than one month: At the end of each month, the lens case (found at any grocery store) should be replaced and a new solution applied. As before, the lenses need to be cleaned again no more than forty-eight hours before wear.

Cosmetics and contact lenses

Cosmetics and contact lenses do not get along well together, but there are ways to make for a compatible union. Educate your patients on these points:

1. Always think of the contact lens first. The patient must place her contact lenses on the eyes *before* any makeup, and she must remove the makeup *before* removing the lenses. This will minimize any chance of makeup coming in contact with the lenses.
2. Avoid "lash-building" mascara. It contains elements that may cause irritation or damage the contact lens.
3. Cover your eyes while using hairspray. Alcohol-free types of hairspray are best, but we still want to train the patient to avoid exposing the lenses to the spray fumes.

Contact lens-wearing schedule

For most typical new contact-lens wearers, the doctor will recommend gradually increasing the wear time each day until the patient is up to a full day. This helps the eye build tolerance to the lens and to the decreased supply of oxygen. A lens-wearing schedule may look like this:

Day 1-2: 8 hours
Day 3-4: 10 hours
Day 5-6: 12 hours
Day 7-8: 14 hours
Day 8-10: 16 hours

So far, the FDA has approved only a very small handful of lenses for sleeping in. A couple of the most common ones are the Night and Day™ brand by Ciba and Purevision™ by Bausch and Lomb. The Night and Day™ brand may be worn for one month, with doctor approval, between removals. The Purevision™ brand may be worn for one week between removals. New ones are coming out quickly, so ask your doctor which ones he prescribes for his patients to sleep in so you can educate your patients on this issue.

The primary reason most contact lenses are not safe to sleep in is their lack of oxygen permeability. The cornea, the front surface of the eye, needs oxygen in order to perform many of its functions, not the least of which is combating infections. With a contact lens on the front of the eye, the amount of oxygen the cornea receives is greatly diminished. Continue this lack of oxygen supply into the nighttime hours, and the eye becomes much more susceptible to serious infections. The FDA has shown that nighttime brands allow a safe amount of oxygen to penetrate to the cornea, even when the eyes are closed.

You will have many patients wearing lenses other then these two brands for extended days. It is in your best interest, and the patients', to educate them on the infection danger of doing this.

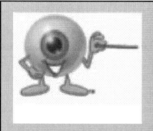

Focus point: In life-threatening conditions, 50 percent of patients do not follow doctor's orders well enough to be effective. For contact lens care, compliance is only 23 percent! Be sure to give written instructions for all lens-care regimens. Your office will likely have these on hand to distribute to your patients.

Finding contact lens specifications

There are literally hundreds of contact lens brands available. In your office, you will find that you routinely use only a handful repeatedly. This helps you remember prices and lens parameters more easily when you order lenses. However, there are bound to be times when a doctor asks you to order a lens you have never heard of. You need a quick-reference guide called *Tyler's Quarterly*® (1-866-664-3788. www.TylersQ.com).

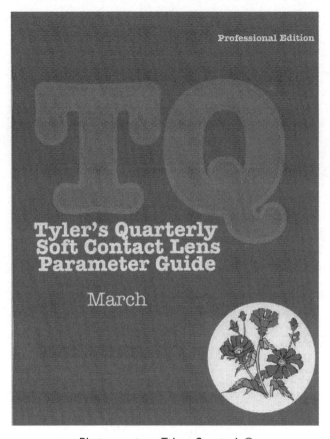

Photo courtesy *Tylers Quarterly®*

Tyler's Quarterly is the bible of contact lenses. It is distributed four times a year to subscribing offices (which includes nearly every office that does any work in contact lenses). Each issue has two main sections. The first is divided into types of contact lenses, such as disposables, colors, and torics. The second section is divided by contact lens manufactures, such as Bausch & Lomb, Ciba, Cooper, Vistakon, and so forth.

The publication lists all the parameters of each lens. When a doctor writes a prescription for a particular brand and lens power, you might discover that the lens power is not available for that brand. When this happens, you should notify the doctor about the next nearest parameters available.

Let us look at the parameters *Tyler's Quarterly* lists for each contact lens:

Vistakon
Order: 1-800-874-5278
Fax: 1-800-456-2733
Consult: 1-877-334-3937
Website: www.ecp.acuvue.com

Multi-Packaged Sphericals - with UV blocker

Parameters →

Manufacturer	Series	Material/ Water Content	Prod. / FDA #	Base Curve (mm)	Diameter (mm)	Power Availability*	Optical Zone	Center Thickness	Disinfection** Method	dK Value	Unit Cost ‡
Silicone Hydrogel											
Vistakon	ACUVUE ADVANCE	galyfilcon A 47% stabilized w/ Hydraclear soft molding 1	2 wk DW	8.3, 8.7	14.0 visibility tint	+0.50 to +8.00, -0.50 to -12.00 (in .50D steps above ±6.00)		.070 (-3.00) .17 (+3.00) (inversion indicator *1 2 3* on front surface)	C & O if reused	60.0	(6 pk) (blister packs)
Note: Oasys approved for therapeutic use; 8.8 BC avail. Jan. 1, 2008	ACUVUE OASYS 1-7day EW	senofilcon A 38% stabilized w/ Hydraclear soft molding 1 Plus Class I UV blocking	2 wk DW	8.4, 8.8	14.0 light blue visibility tint	+0.50 to +8.00, -0.50 to -12.00 (in .50D steps above ±6.00)		.070 (-4.00) .17 (+4.00) (inversion indicator *1 2 3* on front surface)	C & O if reused	103.0	(6 pk) (blister packs)
Disposable Hydrogel											
	ACUVUE 2 (light blue visibility tint)	etafilcon A 58% soft 1-7 day EW or 2 wk DW molding 4	stabilized	8.3, 8.7	14.0	+0.50 to +8.00, -0.50 to -12.00 (in .50D steps above ±6.00)		.084 (-3.00) .17 (+3.00) (inversion indicator *1 2 3* on front surface)	C & O if reused	28.0	(6 pk) (blister packs)
	ACUVUE (light blue visibility tint) (contains inside out *AV* marker)	etafilcon A 58% soft 1 - 7 day EW or 2 wk DW	stabilized molding 4	8.8

8.4

9.1 | 14.0

14.0

14.4 | -0.50 to -11.00 (in .50D steps above -6.00) -0.50 to -9.00 (in .50 D steps above -6.00) +0.50 to +8.00 (in .50D steps above +6.00) | | .07 (-3.00)

.17 (+3.00) | C & O if reused | 28.0 | (6 pk) (blister packs) |
| Note: All Acuvue lenses contain UV blocker & are approved for monovision fitting. | 1•DAY ACUVUE light blue visibility tint Note: New lens design | etafilcon A 58% soft molding, 4 Inversion indicator *1 2 3* on front surface | stabilized | 8.5, 9.0 | 14.2 | +0.50 to +6.00; -0.50 to -12.00 (in 0.50D steps above -6.00) | | .084 (-3.00) .17 (+3.00) | none necessary | 28.0 | (30 pk) |
| | 1•DAY ACUVUE MOIST light blue visibility tint Lacreon moisture rich technology | etafilcon A 58% soft molding, 4 Inversion indicator *1 2 3* on front surface | stabilized | 8.5, 9.0 | 14.2 | +0.50 to +6.00; -0.50 to -12.00 (in 0.50D steps above -6.00) | | .084 (-3.00) .17 (+3.00) | none necessary | 28.0 | (30 pk) |

Multi-Packaged Sphericals - Opaque & Enhancer Tints

Courtesy *Tyler's Quarterly*

1. Manufacturer: This is the name of the company that makes the contact lens. The phone number for the manufacturer is listed for placing orders or for questions.

2. Series: This is the brand name of the contact lens. Just like Ford (the manufacturer) makes many models of cars, contact lens manufactures make many different models of contact lenses.

3. Material/Water Content: This is the material the lens is made of. Each material will have different properties, some with a high content of water and others with a lower content. Some will have a higher propensity for attracting protein deposits, and so forth. It will be up to the doctor to determine which material is best for each patient.

4. Prod.: This is the production method for making the lens. It may make a difference in how well the lens centers on the eye.

5. Base Curve: This is the inside curvature of the contact lens. This determines how "loose" or how "tight" the lens will fit on the eye. If a doctor finds that the contact lens moves too much, or is "too loose," he may decide to steepen the base curve, effectively tightening the lens on the eye. The lower the base curve number, the steeper the curve.

Therefore, a high number base curve would likely move more on an eye than a base curve of a lower value.

6. Diameter: This is the overall diameter of the lens. The bigger the lens, the more stability it may have on the eye—but also the tougher it may be for the patient to insert, especially for those with smaller eyes.

7. Power Availability: This is the range of powers in which this particular contact lens is manufactured.

8. Optic Zone: The power of a contact lens does not span the entire diameter of a lens. Some of the periphery of a lens is just to add mass and stability. This value tells you what size zone in the center of the lens actually carries the prescription. This value may be of use for patients with exceptionally large pupils. In a case such as this, the doctor may wish to use a lens that has a larger optic zone.

9. Center thickness: This is the thickness of the center of the contact lens. The thicker it is, the less oxygen can pass through and may affect comfort..

10. Disinfection Method: This is the manufacturer's suggested disinfection techniques. C stands for chemical disinfection. This is the most common type of disinfection and would include the solutions we discussed earlier in this chapter. H stands for heat disinfection. We do not see this type used very often anymore. O stands for oxidation.

11. dK value: This is a measure of the oxygen permeability of the lens material for a given power. The higher the dK, the greater amount of oxygen capable of penetrating through the lens to the cornea.

12. Unit Cost: This is the wholesale value of the lenses—what your office actually pays for them. Your office will then use a multiple of this, such as 2×, to compute the retail cost for the patient. You will need to learn the multiple your office uses. This column also describes how the lens is supplied, such as a single lens in a vial, a six-pack, or some other combination.

Let us look at a few examples of how *Tyler's Quarterly* may be used.

Example #1: A doctor finds that by using a Vistakon Acuvue 2 contact lens with a base curve of 8.3, the contact lens does not move adequately on the eye. He wishes to know if this lens comes in a *flatter* base curve. How do you find out?

Since we know the manufacturer, Vistakon, and the brand of the lens, Acuvue 2, it would be most efficient to use the second half of *Tylers Quarterly*, which breaks down lenses by manufacturer in alphabetical order. Vistakon would be toward the end of the publication.

Now that we have found Vistakon, look for its Acuvue 2 listing.

Vistakon Order: 1-800-874-5278 Consult: 1-877-334-3937
Fax: 1-800-456-2733 Website: www.ecp.acuvue.com

Multi-Packaged Sphericals - with UV blocker

Manufacturer	Series	Material/ Water Content	Prod. / FDA #	Base Curve (mm)	Diameter (mm)	Power Availability*	Optical Zone	Center Thickness	Disinfection** Method	dK Value	Unit Cost ‡
Silicone Hydrogel											
Vistakon	ACUVUE ADVANCE	galyfilcon A 47% w/ Hydraclear Class I UV blocking	stabilized soft molding 1	8.3, 8.7	14.0 visiblity tint	+0.50 to +8.00, -0.50 to -12.00 (in .50D steps above ±6.00)		.070 (-3.00) .16 (+3.00) (inversion indicator "1 2 3" on front surface)	C & O if reused	60.0	$16.25 (6 pk) (blister packs)
Senofilcon A approved for therapeutic use.	ACUVUE OASYS 1-7day EW	senofilcon A 38% w/ Hydraclear Plus	stabilized soft molding 1 Class I UV blocking visibility tint	8.4, 8.8 2 wk DW	14.0 light blue	Plano (bandage lens) +0.50 to +8.00 -0.50 to -12.00 (in .50D steps above ±6.00)		.070 (-3.00) .147 (+3.00) (inversion indicator "1 2 3" on front surface)	C & O if reused	103.0	$20.25 (6 pk) (blister packs)
Disposable Hydrogel											
	ACUVUE 2 (light blue visibility tint)	etafilcon A 58% 1-7 day EW or 2 wk DW	stabilized soft molding 4	8.3, 8.7	14.0	+0.50 to +8.00, -0.50 to -12.00 (in .50D steps above ±6.00)		.084 (-3.00) .17 (+3.00) (inversion indicator "1 2 3" on front surface)	C & O if reused	28.0	$13.50 (6 pk) (blister packs)

Base curve options

Courtesy *Tyler's Quarterly*

Slide your finger across to the Base Curve column, and you will see that Acuvue 2 comes in an 8.3 and an 8.7 base curve. Therefore, the doctor's goal of finding a flatter lens, the 8.7 base curve, is possible while keeping the patient in the Acuvue 2 brand.

Let us look at another example of the use of *Tyler's Quarterly*. Scan across the Acuvue 2 listing to the final column labeled "Unit Cost."

We see that the wholesale cost of this lens is $13.50 and that the lens comes supplied as a six-pack. Each office may use a different multiple for calculating retail cost, but let us assume your office uses a multiple of 2×. Therefore, you would charge the patient $27.00 per six-pack box ($13.50 × 2). You will need to find out from your manager what multiple you use for calculating contact lens prices.

Once you use *Tyler's Quarterly* a handful of times, you will become very efficient at finding lenses.

Chapter 6 test

1. What are the advantages and disadvantages of soft contact lenses vs. rigid contact lenses?

2. What is a *greenie* used for?

3. Do cleaners disinfect?

4. What should a patient do with a lens she will store for more than a month without wear?

5. What publication do you turn to when you want to find contact lens parameters and prices?

CHAPTER 7

Ocular Conditions and Related Visual Symptoms

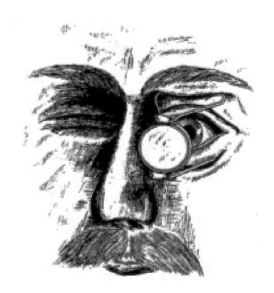

O **NLY** one thing is more frustrating to an optician than having a patient come into the office and complain he is not seeing well with his new glasses. That is spending an hour with the patient, checking that everything is OK with the way the glasses were made, and then having the patient tell you that he has macular degeneration and asking whether that affects his vision.

Glasses cannot save the world, and they certainly cannot get patients to see any better than an eye condition allows them to see. Often patients expect miracles from their glasses. Their doctor should thoroughly explain realistic expectations before patients leave the room, but patients often forget this conversation by the time they pick up their glasses. The patients wonder why street signs are still difficult to read, and usually they blame you.

This chapter is devoted to helping you recognize the symptoms associated with the most common visual conditions so you may better separate *eyeglass* problems from *eyeball* problems.

Cataracts: Hey, doc, I'm livin' in a fog!

Cataracts happen. They happen to everyone eventually, and they will happen to you, too, one day. Usually starting in a person's mid-60s, cataracts are a clouding and browning of the lens inside the eye. When we are born, our lens is crystal clear, like a fine-quality diamond. However, as we age, this lens slowly becomes cloudy and discolors. When this happens, we call it a cataract.

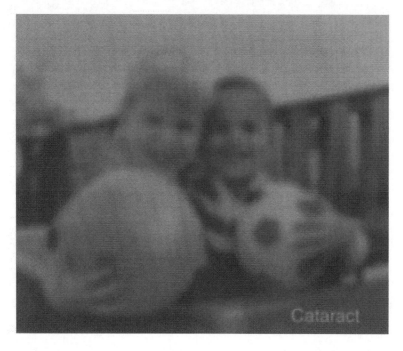

Simulation of vision with a cataract (Courtesy: National Eye Institute, National Institutes of Health)

Early cataracts may not have any symptoms at all. However, as they progress, patients will increasingly complain of a "film over my eyes," nighttime starbursts around lights, or generally "foggy" vision.

Once vision is reduced to the 20/40 level (a common minimum vision needed to pass a driving vision test), it is usually time to have the cataracts removed. This has evolved into a routine outpatient surgery that most ophthalmologists are able to do in their office. The procedure takes approximately twenty minutes with the patient fully awake. Once the doctor removes the cataract, he replaces it with an intraocular lens implant.

Prior to the development of these implants, following cataract surgery, patients would need to wear thick "cataract glasses" to compensate for the removed lens. You may recall that the lens inside the eye is responsible for much of the refracting power, so if it is removed without a new lens to replace it, glasses must make up the lost power. The new synthetic lenses have made the old thick glasses unnecessary, though most patients still need to wear some type of glasses after the surgery to obtain their best possible vision.

Cataracts rarely cause any harm to the eye; they only keep the patient from seeing as well as they otherwise could without the cataracts. Therefore, the removal of a cataract is rarely a medical necessity. Typically, it is the patient's discretion as to when to have it removed. One patient may say, "Get this cataract out of me as soon as you can! I want to see better," whereas another patient may say, "No way! No one is going to be cutting on my eye until it gets a lot worse!" And both responses are usually perfectly acceptable.

Macular Degeneration

Macular degeneration can be a visually devastating eye condition. It is the number one cause of legal blindness in adults over the age of 60 in the United States. About 40 percent of people over the age of 75 have the condition. The macula is a very small part of the eye, but the most important part, for it gives us our fine-detail vision. Whenever you look at an object, it is the macula the object's image falls upon. When this degenerates, the end stage of the disease is a black spot within the line of vision. The only thing the patient has left is peripheral vision.

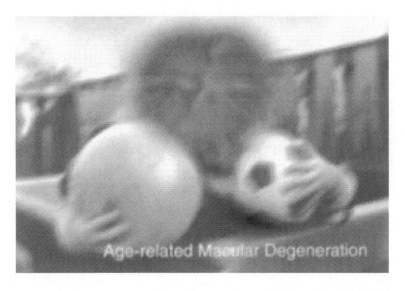

Macular degeneration simulation (Courtesy: National Eye Institute, National Institutes of Health)

Early in the onset, patients may report simply a slightly blurry spot in their vision or that straight lines, such as door jams, appear wavy. As the condition advances, this blurry spot becomes a dark spot. Patients often report that when they look at your face, all they see is your hair and clothing (in their peripheral vision).

Macular degeneration has two stages of advancement. In the first stage, called the *dry stage*, the macula undergoes only structural changes. Although people can progress to legally blind in the dry stage, patients often consider the dry stage to be the mild form of macular degeneration. But as it progresses, blood vessels under the macula leak, causing hemorrhages. This is the *wet stage*, which is nearly always visually debilitating because of the large amount of swelling and scar tissue left behind. Patients often think of the wet and dry type of macular degeneration as two distinctly separate diseases, when they are simply two ends of the disease spectrum.

Risk factors for macular degeneration include the following:

- **Smoking.** Studies have shown smokers have twice the risk for macular degeneration of non-smokers.
- **Obesity.** Being obese is linked with more rapid progression of macular degeneration.

- **Race.** Caucasians are more likely to have macular degeneration than other races.
- **Family history.** A family history of macular degeneration increases your risk for the condition.
- **Gender.** Women are at greater risk than men.
- **General health.** Those with high blood pressure or high cholesterol are at higher risk.
- **Poor diet.** Those with diets lacking adequate levels of fruits and vegetables or with excessive saturated fats have higher incidences of macular degeneration.

There is no cure for macular degeneration. Lasers and injections used often to slow its progress at the wet stage, but as of today, there is no way to reverse its damage. There are many studies lately into nutritional means to slow its progress, such as multiple vitamins or other dietary supplements such as Lutein, but none of these therapies has been shown to help patients regain the sight they have already lost from the disease.

Diabetic Retinopathy:

Diabetes is an increasingly prevalent condition in the United States. With diabetes, the body is unable to adequately control the sugar levels in the blood. Long term, this leads to a weakening of the blood vessel walls and hemorrhages within the eye. Additionally, as the blood sugar varies, changes can take place in the shape of the lens that can drastically alter a person's prescription. For these reasons, a routine eye exam will often lead to a diagnosis of diabetes.

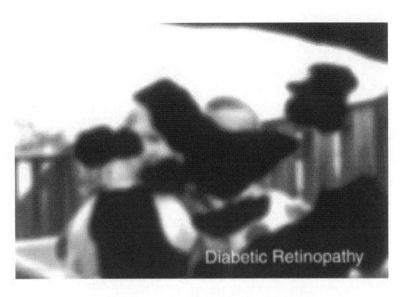

Simulation of vision with diabetic retinopathy
(Courtesy: National Eye Institute, National Institutes of Health)

The hemorrhaging in the eye typically causes the visual loss associated with diabetes. Most diabetics, after ten years, will have some mild hemorrhages within the eye; but with good blood-sugar control, these hemorrhages are small, do not cause harm, and resolve within a few weeks without any visual complications.

Larger hemorrhages that occur in the area of the macula may cause severe vision loss. They leave behind a scar or permanent distortion to the retinal tissue. Often, these large hemorrhages and their resulting swelling of the retina require treatment with laser therapy. The laser, however, has its own drawback. Although it can help reduce the swelling and prevent some future hemorrhages, it also leaves behind a scar of its own. Often, patients report that their vision was made worse by the laser treatment, and sometimes they are right. However, what the patient fails to realize in these cases is that the treatment may have prevented even more vision loss in the future.

Glaucoma

Glaucoma is an eye disease in which the pressure of fluid inside the eye damages the optic nerve. The point at which that pressure causes harm is different for everyone. Some people have a nerve of steel, and even high pressure will cause no harm to the nerve. Other people's nerves, however, may be susceptible to even very low pressure. You may see the Intraocular Pressure (IOP) measurement recorded in the patient's medical chart. Typically, the pressure will be between 10–20 mmHg; however, in glaucoma, the pressure often rises well above 20.

Early in the course of glaucoma, there are no symptoms at all. In most cases, the increase in pressure associated with glaucoma will not cause any headaches, blurred vision, or other symptoms. Patients will often come into an office complaining of headaches around the eyes and are afraid it is a sign of glaucoma. More often than not, however, this is simply a sign of sinus congestion. Ironically, patients who never come in for an eye exam because they perceive that "everything is just fine" are the ones who have silently progressing glaucoma.

Glaucoma must become moderately advanced before any visual symptoms will emerge. This is what makes glaucoma so dangerous and prevents patients from seeking eyecare sooner in its progression. As the optic nerve becomes increasingly damaged, the person's peripheral visual field becomes constricted in a tunnel-like fashion. The visual field will likely be tested by the doctor about every six months on a machine called an *automated perimeter*. The test is much like a video game. Patients look into a large dome and press a button whenever they see a small light appear in their peripheral vision. The instrument documents what lights are not seen, and a printout is made showing these points. Glaucoma will create a very characteristic pattern of misses.

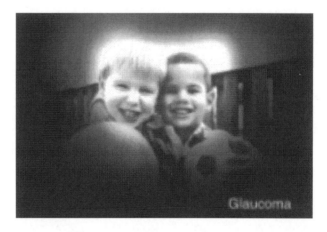

Simulation of vision with glaucoma (Courtesy: National Eye Institute, National Institutes of Health)

The treatment for glaucoma is typically an eye drop taken once or twice a day that lowers the fluid pressure in the eye. Depending on the type of drop, it either reduces the production of fluid in the eye or increases its outflow from the eye. In most cases, this eye drop is all that is needed to keep the pressure in the eye low enough to prevent further nerve damage. Occasionally, however, even multiple eye drops are not enough, and surgery is then required to help reduce the pressure further.

Floaters

The word "floaters" describes an eye condition doctors hear patients complain about often; fortunately, however, floaters by themselves cause no harm to the eye. They are often a byproduct of the vitreous, the viscous fluid inside the eye that helps maintain the eye's shape. Occasionally, this fluid will clump in areas. If one of these clumps happens to form or pass by the patient's line of sight through the center of the eye, the patient will report seeing a shadow. We call this a floater. The dissolving of an embryonic blood vessel within the eye cavity can also leave behind particles seen to the patient as floaters. This is a very normal process.

Floaters come in many shapes and sizes. Some patients may report seeing little gnats flying about in front of their head; other patients may report that it looks like a large cat laying on the floor or "strings" floating in the air. A new onset of floaters, associated with flashing lights, or a change in the appearance of their floaters, should always be reported to a doctor for evaluation to ensure it is not something more serious.

Although there are 1,000-page textbooks devoted to all the things that can go wrong with an eye, these are the most common ones you will run into in your office. With a good grasp of your patients' medical history, you should be able to explain to them why they are not able to see those street signs a mile down the freeway like they used to and save the doctor from a time-consuming prescription recheck office visit.

Oftentimes, new glasses may actually make a condition, especially macular degeneration, more noticeable for the patient. Let us look at an example of how this can happen. A patient sees his eye doctor complaining his vision is not as clear as it used to be. The doctor measures his vision at 20/80. With new glasses, the doctor is able to get the patient to see 20/50. The reason the patient cannot be corrected to 20/20 is found to be macular degeneration. When the patient picks up his glasses, he is measured as seeing 20/50, yet complains that he saw better with his old glasses. "I have a large smudge on my glasses with these new ones that I can't clean away!" the patient states. What happened?

The patient never noticed his central blind spot from macular degeneration with his old glasses, because with the blurriness created by wearing an old prescription, even his peripheral vision was blurry. This masked some of the central blur created by the macular degeneration. The new glasses cleared the peripheral vision enough to highlight the central macular degeneration. Similar to excavating a fossil, you do not see the bone (macular degeneration) until the dirt (refractive error) is cleared away. Glasses may occasionally clear away the dirt to reveal the underlying condition. This will be discussed further in the next chapter.

Summary of eye conditions and related visual complaints

Cataracts:
1. Dimness of colors
2. Blurry/Foggy (may masquerade as incorrect Rx)
3. Increased glare, especially at night

Macular Degeneration:
1. Straight lines appear wavy (patients often refer to bent door frames)
2. Images disappear when focused upon (may masquerade as a central scratch in the lens)
3. Blur/Fog

Diabetic Retinopathy:
1. Vision fluctuates throughout day or week
2. Areas of dimness in periphery and poor nighttime vision (after laser treatment)

Glaucoma:
1. Dimness of vision
2. Colors seem less vibrant (in later stages)
3. Tunnel vision (in late stages)

Floaters:
1. "Strings," "gnats" or other household objects in vision.
2. Shadows

Chapter 7 test

1. What are three symptoms of cataracts?
2. What are three symptoms of macular degeneration?
3. What is the most likely explanation for patients complaining of seeing "strings" in their vision?
4. Why may a person with glaucoma not seek out treatment?

CHAPTER 8

Special Cases—Recognizing Potential Pitfalls

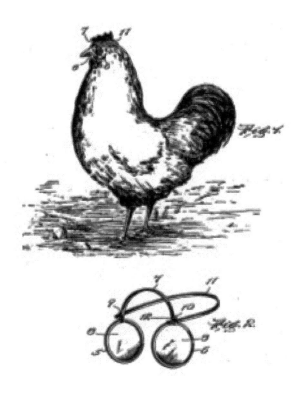

THERE are bound to be scenarios that arise in your career as an optician only on infrequent occasions. This chapter will try to prepare you for those occasions. As a new optician in training, you would probably be happy to remember half of what has been discussed so far. However, by learning how to deal with the following special cases, you can appear to be wise beyond your years!

Anisometropia

Anisometropia is a condition in which the two eyes have a need for drastically different prescriptions (>2.00 diopters of difference). One of two factors can cause this: 1) the patient is simply born this way; or 2) cataract surgery resulted in the different prescriptions.

Initially, the cosmetic appearance of the lenses may come to mind. If one lens is higher power than the other, it will also be thicker and more unsightly. This cosmetic factor must be addressed in order to make the patient's *spouse* happy. Since the cosmetic appearance of the lenses is typically the first thing to come to the optician's mind, the second and more visually debilitating condition is often overlooked.

This second result of anisometropia is *aniseikonia,* the nausea the patient will feel if something isn't done to correct the image size difference the two eyes are receiving. This factor must be addressed to make the *patient* happy. If the brain receives an image from a +2.00D lens in one eye and from a +5.00D lens in the other eye, the sizes of the images will be different, and the brain will have a hard time fusing these two images. A queasy patient will likely return to you saying that the glasses are making her sick.

The third result of anisometropia is induced prism, in which the patient looks off-center, resulting in double vision. Recall that a lens can be thought of as two prisms placed together, and that images are displaced toward the base of the prism. Remember also Prentice's Rule, which showed that 1) the further off-axis a person looks, the greater the prismatic effect; and 2) the greater the lens power, the greater the prismatic effect from looking off-axis.

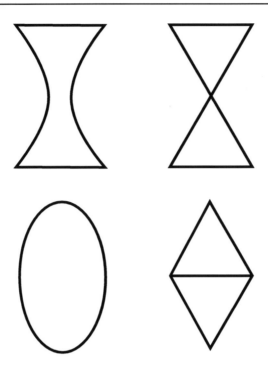

Similarity of eyeglass lenses (left) with prisms (right)

Looking "off-center" effectively is the same as looking through a prism.

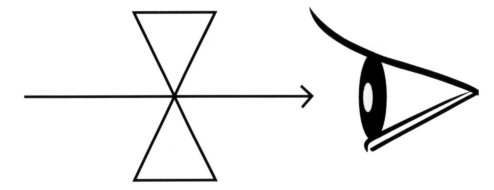

Looking through the optical center of the lens

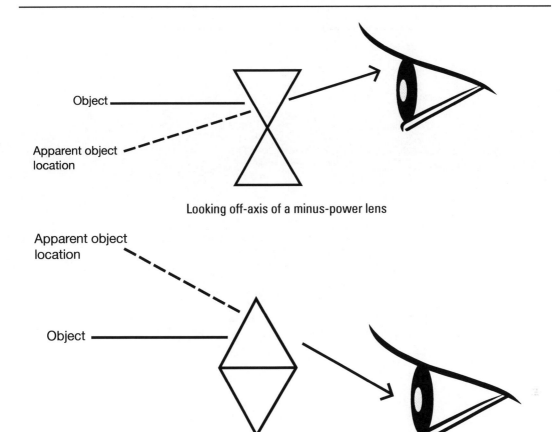

Looking off-axis of a minus-power lens

Looking off-axis of a plus-power lens

As long as the prescriptions in each eye are close, the amount of prism induced in each lens by looking off-axis is relatively equal (Prentice's Rule). This allows the induced prism to be small enough to cause no noticeable prismatic effect to the wearer. However, imagine the effect when the two prescriptions are drastically different.

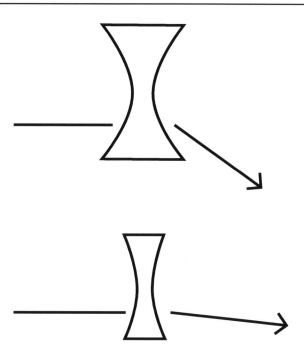

Different lens powers create different prismatic effects

The above illustration shows why if the patient looks off-axis in glasses that are of drastically different powers, one eye will experience a far greater prismatic effect than the other eye (recall Prentice's Rule). This creates a net imbalance for which the eye muscles cannot compensate, and double vision results. This effect will occur in every direction off-center the eye looks, whether it is up, down, left, or right.

So now that we know the three things that anisometropia creates, what can we do to correct them? Keep in mind your average optician will be lucky to know how to correct two of the three, so if you can correct all three, you will be far ahead of your peers on day one!

The cosmetic factor

The best way to minimize a difference in thickness between the two lenses, and therefore improve the cosmetic appearance, is to use a high-index material. By thinning both lenses, the difference in thickness between them appears more subtle. The difference in thickness between a +3.00 and +5.00 is much more pronounced in conventional plastic than in polycarbonate or some other high-index plastic.

Additionally, selecting a small frame helps prevent the difference in edge thickness from becoming too noticeable. When lenses are ordered from a lab, they come in a large "blank" which is then cut down to the frame size. The more of the blank that needs to be cut, the thinner the edges will be.

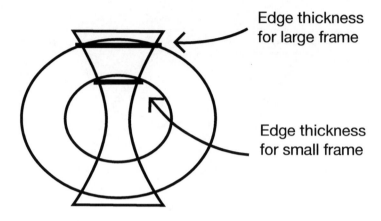

A small frame size will create a thinner lens edge. This means less off-axis prismatic effect and a more attractive lens.

The nausea factor

Aniseikonia, the feeling of nausea that comes from wearing glasses with dramatically different prescriptions in each eye, comes from the magnification difference each eye is receiving. To minimize the nausea, therefore, you must minimize the different image size each lens is creating. Lenses of different powers will always provide a slightly different image size to each eye, but there are ways to minimize the effect.

One of the most simple and cost-efficient ways to accomplish this is to specify on the order to make the base curves and center thickness of the lenses as equal as possible (given the power difference). This will be a very effective one-two punch. Equalizing the center thickness will mean making the lower-power lens a little thicker than it otherwise would have to be. Making the lenses close to the same thickness will aid in minimizing the magnification difference, and, therefore, the nausea.

Making the lens aspheric will also minimize the aniseikonia. Recall that making a lens aspheric will flatten the lens; this will both help make the lenses closer to the same thickness as well as help minimize "off-axis" image-size differences due to peripheral curvature differences.

The double vision factor

In a single-vision lens, patients can simply move their heads in the direction they want to look. Although it may require more head movement than is desired, it is possible to keep your sight through the optical center of the lens whether looking in the distance or reading.

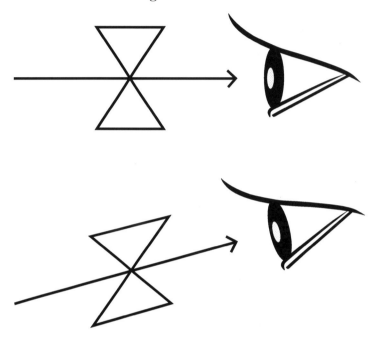

A single-vision lens wearer can tilt his head downward to maintain sight through the optic center lens.

Now visualize a bifocal wearer. A bifocal *forces* the wearer to look "off-center" in order to appreciate the reading help of the bifocal

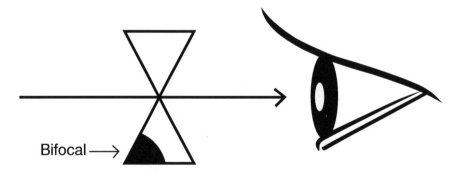

A bifocal wearer in distance gaze.

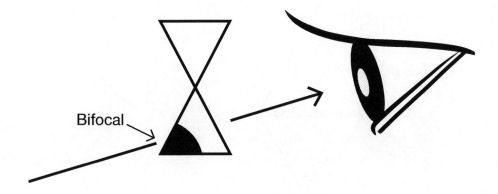

A bifocal wearer in reading gaze. The patient must look off-axis to use the bifocal section of the lenses.

If there is a high amount of anisometropia, the patient will see double every time she tries to read due to the different prismatic effect caused by looking off-center. For example, let's assume the right eye is myopic and needs a minus-power lens …

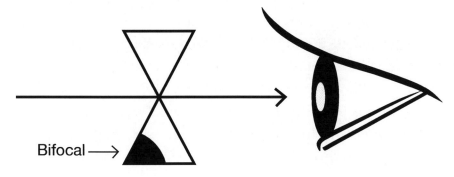

The base-down effect created by looking through the bifocal of a minus-power lens.

In addition, suppose the left eye is hyperopic and needs a plus power lens …

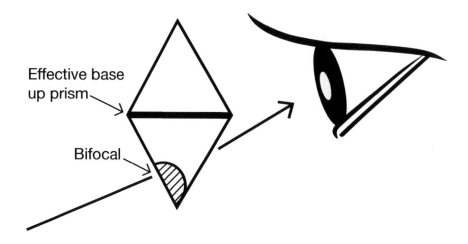

Effective base up prism

Bifocal

As you can see in this extreme case of anisometropia, the right eye is experiencing a base-down prism effect while the left eye is experiencing a base-up prism effect. This certainly will create double vision for this patient. However, this can happen even in less extreme cases. For example, if both eyes are nearsighted, but one eye requires a -1.00 lens and the other eye requires a -4.00 lens, the base-down prism created by the difference in edge thickness between these two lenses could be enough to create double vision for the patient.

Slab-off is used in these cases when there is a high amount of anisometropia, usually greater than 2.00 diopters, in the 90° axis of the lenses, and the patient needs a multifocal lens (or any lens that will require the patient to look off-axis). Slab-off is *offsetting* prism ground into the lens at the level of the bifocal to counteract the prism induced by the anisometropia. The only visual clue that slab-off is present in a pair of glasses is a faint line extending the entire length of the lens just above the bifocal line. Unlike prescribed prism, which as we know is usually split between the two eyes, slab-off is placed on just one of the lenses. A patient will typically be willing to overlook this slight cosmetic drawback because it eliminates double vision.

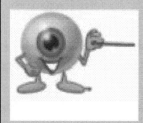

Focus point: In cases of anisometropia, in which the power difference is greater than 2.00 diopters between the two eyes in the 90° axis and the patient needs a bifocal, always specify *slab-off* on the order.

Slab-off can be placed only on the inferior part of the lens with a bifocal. Although this is wonderful at reducing double vision in downward gaze, the patient will still see double if looking off to the side or up. Keep in mind, there is nothing about the bifocal itself causing the double vision; the double vision is the result of having to look off-axis with a pair of lenses of different thicknesses. Imagine patients with high amounts of anisometropia who have unusual visual demands as part of their job, such as an airline pilot who has to look upward to see gauges, a mechanic who gets into some awkward position, or any other occupation that requires the person to look away from the very center of the lens. These patients will have the same double vision in up-gaze or side-gaze as they would have in down-gaze without slab-off.

To minimize this as much as possible, try to direct these patients into small frames. The further off-axis the patients look when they have anisometropia, the greater the prismatic effect (and therefore double vision) will be. By having the patients wear a small frame, it limits how far off-axis they can look. This encourages them to turn their head to what they want to see and keeps them closer to the optical center of the lens.

You may recall this illustration from earlier in the chapter. It illustrates how the further off-axis you look, the more prism that is induced from lens thickness changes, and explains why small frames work so well in these cases to keep the patient centered..

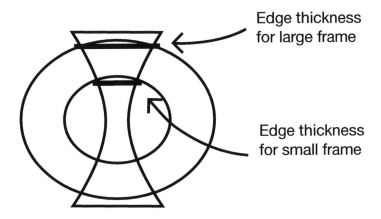

A smaller frame minimizes the off-axis prism induced in each lens by minimizing edge thickness.

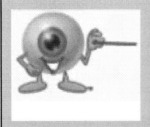

Focus point: When presented with a patient with anisometropia, always lean toward smaller frames. This will accomplish two goals: 1) It will make the lenses cosmetically more appealing by minimizing the apparent difference in lens thickness; and 2) it will minimize the distance the patient can look off axis, thereby minimizing the off-axis prismatic effects.

Fortunately, as the optician, you do not generally need to calculate the amount of offsetting prism that is needed or which eye it needs to be placed on. Simply recognize that slab-off is needed if the prescription difference is greater than 2.00 diopters in each eye and request it on the order. The laboratory will do all the calculations. However, it is a good idea to be familiar with the calculations the lab will use in determining the amount of slab-off that is needed. Recalling the Prentice Rule formula for calculating prism from a previous chapter will help you see how slab-off works.

Here is a slab-off example:

A patient has a prescription of +1.00 DS in the right eye and +5.00 DS in the left with a +2.00 bifocal. What amount of slab-off is required to keep this patient from seeing double when she reads?

Recall the equation: Prism = Power × Decentration (in centimeters)
We assume that a patient will look downward 1 cm to use a bifocal.

Therefore, for the right eye, the induced Prism = 1.00 × 1cm = 1 diopter
And for the left eye, the induced Prism = 5.00 × 1cm = 5 diopters

Is the induced prism in the base-up or base-down direction in each eye? Recall that a lens is simply two prisms placed together. For a plus lens, the two bases of the prisms are together in the center.

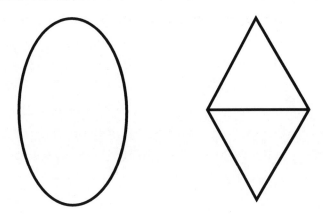

A plus lens (left) is the same as two prisms with bases together in the center (right)

By looking downward from the optical center of the lens, the base (the thick part of the prism) will be above the patient's line of sight. Therefore, the patient will experience *base-up* prism in each eye since each eye is a plus lens.

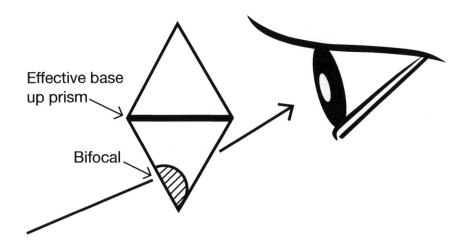

Base-up effect from looking through the bifocal of a plus-power lens

So now we know that the patient will experience 1 diopter of base-up prism in the right eye and 5 diopters of base-up prism in the left. What is the net effect? Recall from our chapter on prism that when measuring vertical prism, the net effect is the difference between what the two eyes experience (horizontal prism, by comparison, is measured by taking the sum of each lens's prism). So if the right eye is experiencing 1 diopter base-up and the left eye 5 diopters base-up, the net effect is therefore 4 diopters of vertical prism (5-1). This can be expressed as either 4 base-up in the left eye or 4 base-down in the right. *A pair of eyes is typically able to overcome only about 0.5 to 1.0 diopter of vertical prism before the patient sees double.* Therefore, in this case, the patient definitely will see double when reading unless compensating slab-off prism is used.

Four diopters of slab-off prism, therefore, will be ground by the laboratory onto a lens to provide 4 diopters of compensating prism. Which lens will end up with the compensating slab-off prism depends on the type of slab-off the lab uses. Conventional slab-off is base-up. Therefore, in order for conventional slab-off (base-up prism) to be compensating for a prism imbalance, it must be placed on the lens causing the most base-down prism effect. *This will always be the most minus- or least plus-power lens.*

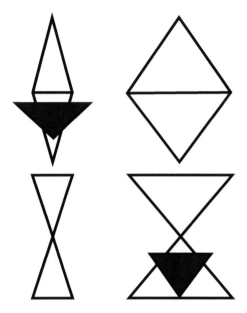

A schematic illustration of slab-off. In plus-power prescriptions (top), slab-off is placed on the least plus lens. This adds base-up prism to the lens that has the least base-up effect to make it equal in prismatic effect to the other lens. In minus-power prescriptions (bottom), slab-off placed on the most minus-power lens will add base-up prism to the lens that has the most base-down effect, thereby neutralizing this excessive base-down prism effect.

To make things complicated, some labs will use *reverse* slab-off. The principle is the same, except that the compensating ground-in prism is base-down. Therefore, in order for *reverse* slab-off (base-down prism) to be compensating, it is placed on the lens causing the most base-up prism effect. *This will always be the least minus- or most plus-power lens.*

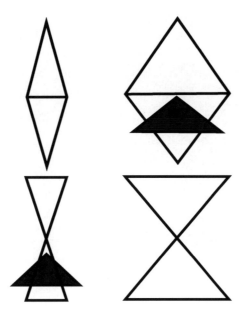

A schematic illustration of reverse slab-off. In plus-power prescriptions (top), reverse slab-off is placed on the most plus lens. This adds base-down prism to the lens that has the most base-up effect, thereby neutralizing this excessive base-up effect. In minus-power prescriptions (bottom), reverse slab-off placed on the least minus-power lens will add base-down prism to the lens that has the least base-down effect, thereby making the prismatic effect more equal to the other lens.

It may now be apparent to you why we care about the power difference only in the 90° axis of the lenses when considering a slab-off. When patients look downward through the bifocal, they are following the 90-degree (vertical) path of the lens. When dealing with a spherical lens, as in the previous example, it makes no difference which way the patient looks off-center; the power is the same. However, when dealing with an astigmatism-correcting lens, there *is* a difference due to the change in power of each axis. How, then, do we calculate the power in the 90° axis in someone with an astigmatism lens to determine if the person needs slab-off? Let us look at an example:

A patient's prescription is

OD:	-2.00 – 1.00 × 180
OS:	-3.00 – 2.00 × 180
Add:	+2.50

You may think there is only a 1.00D difference between the two eyes if you look only at the sphere powers. However, the cylinder powers throw a wrench into this assumption. In order to determine the power in each axis, first place your finger over the cylinder number. Doing this for the right eye (OD) leaves visible the power of -2.00 and the axis of 180. This tells you the power in the 180° axis is -2.00D.

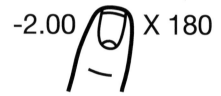

Now remove your finger and add the sphere and the cylinder powers together. This gives you -3.00 (-2.00 + -1.00). This power will be 90 degrees away from the axis, placing it at axis 90° (90° away from 180° is 90°). **Therefore, we now know that the power in the right eye in the 90° axis is -3.00D.**

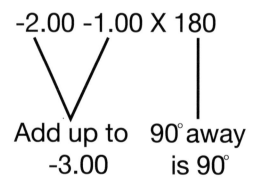

To help you visualize what 90 degrees away from any axis looks like, it helps to remember the axis dial.

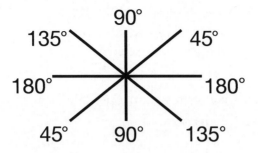

The Axis Dial

Now let us do the same for the left eye. Place your finger over the cylinder and what do you find? That the power in the 180° axis is -3.00D. Now remove your finger and add the sphere and the cylinder powers together and what do you get? A power of -5.00D. What do we know about this power? That it will be 90° from the first, placing it at 90° (90° from 180° is 90°).

Now that we know the power in the 90° axis for the right eye is -3.00D and for the left eye is -5.00D, does this patient need slab-off? Yes! The difference between the two eyes is 2.00D, meeting our 2.00D criteria, so you will want to specify slab-off on the order form.

Here's another example, this time in plus-cylinder form.

Patient's prescription is:
OD: -3.00 + 3.00 × 170
OS: -3.00 + 0.50 × 010

Does this patient need slab-off?

To start, you can usually round the axis off to the nearest 180° or 90° to make your math easy and still end up with a valid answer. So in this case, since axis 170° and 010° are both closer to 180° than 90°, we will assume the axis is 180° in both cases.

What is the power in the 90° axis in the right eye? Cover the cylinder power with your finger and you see that axis 180° has a power of -3.00D. We, however, want 90°, so now add the sphere and cylinder powers together and this will get you 90° away from the 180°, at 90°. Adding the two powers together gives us 0.00 or Plano (-3.00 + +3.00) at 90°. Doing the same for the left eye gives us a power in the 90° of -2.50D (-3.00 + +0.50).

So what is the difference in power in the 90°? The difference between 0.00D and 2.50D is 2.50D. This is greater than our 2.00D criteria for slab-off, so this patient does need slab-off ordered.

What if the axis is exactly between axis 90° and 180°, such as axis 45° or 135°. How do you then determine the power in the 90° axis since it is the same distance from 90° as it is 180°? The previous method we used obviously will not work here. Fortunately, these cases are very rare. You will find the majority of prescriptions have an axis within 20-degrees from the 90° or 180°. However, when a very oblique axis does present itself, a simple rule to follow is to add half of the cylinder to the sphere. The result is the power in both the 90 and 180 axis.

For example, what is the power in the 90° axis in a lens with a prescription of

-3.00 + 2.00 × 135

Adding half the cylinder (+1.00) to the sphere (-3.00) we find a power of -2.00D is at both the 90° and 180° axis. PhDs in optics would say that this is not 100-percent accurate. However, for the purposes of determining the need for slab-off in a clinical setting it is a very useful rule-of-thumb.

Although you will not need to calculate the *amount* of slab-off prism to grind into the lens, because that is a lab job, you will need to recognize *when* slab-off is needed. This knowledge will keep your patients happily seeing single images when they use their bifocals to read.

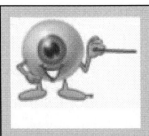

Focus Point:

Things to remember when presented with
anisometropia

1. Equalize the base curve
2. Equalize the center thickness
3. Steer the patient toward a smaller frame
4. Specify slab-off on the order if there is more
   than a 2.00D difference in power in the 90°
   axis and the patient needs a bifocal, trifocal, or
   progressive.

There are a few ways to solve vertical imbalance problems caused by anisometropia without the use of slab-off:

1. Separate distance and reading glasses. This provides the patient with glasses that do not require the patient to look off-axis as a bifocal does.
2. Raise the bifocal seg height. Although this may place the bifocal line in the way of the patient's distance vision, it will allow the patient not to have to look as far off-axis to use the bifocal, and therefore less prism effect will be created. Due to the bifocal line interference with distance vision, this should not be your first choice to solve the issue of anisometropia-induced double vision. Slab-off or separate distance and reading glasses are much better options.
3. Use contact lenses. A *monovision* contact lens fitting could be used. This is when one eye is fit with distance-vision correction and the other eye is fit with a near-vision correction. Another option is to correct both eyes for distance with the contact lenses, but then the patient will need to use reading glasses for any close work.

The Fossil in the Sand

One eye condition can often mask another. Fixing one problem can often reveal a Pandora's box of problems you were not expecting. Let us look at a few examples so you will know how to explain such scenarios to patients.

Example: The cataract patient with macular degeneration

A patient with cataracts, as we learned in a previous chapter, will see a fog-like appearance to everything. Both peripheral and central vision will be compromised. Suppose that you have been seeing a cataract patient for several years, and each year as the cataract progresses, the patient's vision slowly becomes foggier. This patient, as you see in her chart, also has moderately advanced macular degeneration.

One day, the patient comes back to you and exclaims, "The doctor took out my cataracts, and now I can see so much better!" After she expresses her excitement, she tells you the real reason she came in was to have her glasses cleaned. She feels as if there is a black smudge in the center of both lenses. Upon inspection, you find the glasses to be perfectly clean. What is the patient experiencing?

Recall that macular degeneration creates a central blur or blind spot in a patient's vision. In our patient's case, the fog created by the cataracts was hiding the visual effects from the macular degeneration. Once the cataracts were removed, the macular degeneration could be appreciated in all its glory. Similar to digging through sand to uncover a fossil, a cataract (the sand) can hide the underlying macular degeneration (the bones). Remove the sand, and the bones are much easier to see!

Example: The glaucoma and the glasses

An elderly man has gone four years since his last glasses prescription update. In the meantime, he has been treated for glaucoma, which, as you see in his chart, is much worse in his left eye than his right. He saw his doctor for new glasses and is now seeing you to have the prescription filled.

When the man picks up his glasses, he states, "The right eye is great, but I still can't see well in the left eye!" You check out the glasses and find everything is as prescribed. At this point, you can send the patient back to the referring doctor for a reexamination of his prescription, or you can go to the chart to refresh your memory that the patient has advanced glaucoma in the left eye. (If you work independently from an eye doctor, you can call the doctor's office to ask if there is any reason one eye would not see as well as another.)

In this case, the decreased vision from the outdated glasses prescription (the sand) was masking the vision loss from the glaucoma (the underlying fossil). Although new glasses were able to help the right eye with mild glaucoma, the left eye, with advanced glaucoma, was beyond the help that glasses could provide alone.

The average optician in this case would have set the patient up with another appointment with the doctor to have the prescription rechecked. However, you, the enlightened optician, now know to check the chart or call the doctor first to find any alternative possibility for the decreased vision.

Chapter 8 test

1. At what level of anisometropia do symptoms typically appear?
2. What is the solution to anisometropia greater then 2.0D in the 90° axis when the patient needs a bifocal?
3. What four things can you do to minimize the effects of anisometropia in any patient, whether or not the patient needs a bifocal?
4. When slab-off is prescribed, on which lens is it applied?
5. Why might cataract surgery make macular degeneration symptoms more noticeable?

CHAPTER 9

Lab Knowledge for the Non-Lab Optician

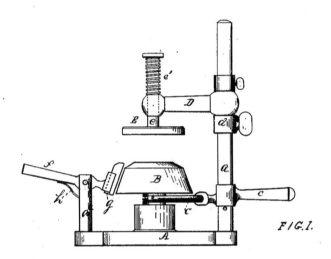

FIG.1.

THERE are opticians and ophthalmic lab technicians unfortunately rarely cross paths. This is unfortunate. Dispensing opticians who know what goes on behind the lab door not only communicate with patients with more authority, it also helps you ask the right questions when calling your lab for assistance. This helps prevents problems from arising both in the lab and on your dispensing floor.

This chapter will discuss the three key processes a dispensing optician should to know about what goes on in the lab. 1) Lens fabrication 2) Troubleshooting 3) Lens tinting tips. The purpose of this is not to make you an expert lab technician, but rather to help you become better versed in understanding what goes on behind the lab door.

THE LIFECYCLE OF OPHTHALMIC LENSES

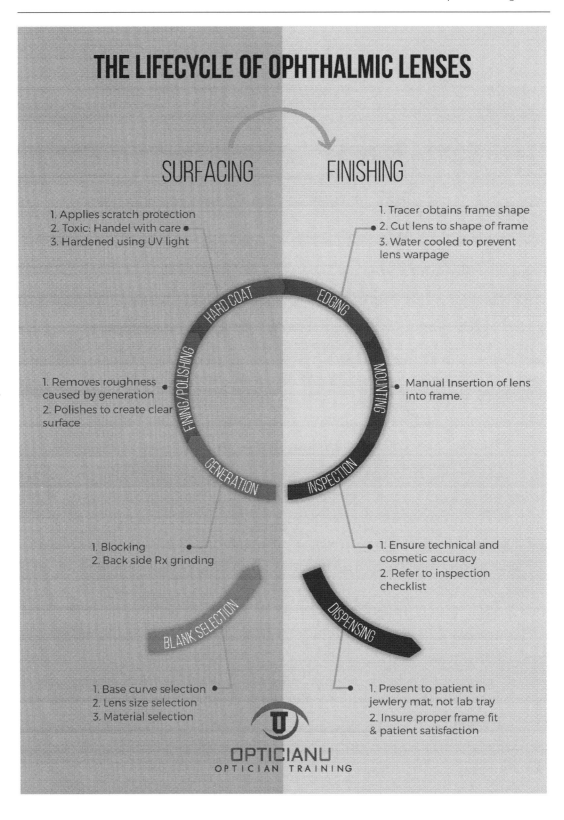

SURFACING

HARD COAT
1. Applies scratch protection
2. Toxic: Handel with care
3. Hardened using UV light

FINING/POLISHING
1. Removes roughness caused by generation
2. Polishes to create clear surface

GENERATION
1. Blocking
2. Back side Rx grinding

BLANK SELECTION
1. Base curve selection
2. Lens size selection
3. Material selection

FINISHING

EDGING
1. Tracer obtains frame shape
2. Cut lens to shape of frame
3. Water cooled to prevent lens warpage

MOUNTING
Manual Insertion of lens into frame.

INSPECTION
1. Ensure technical and cosmetic accuracy
2. Refer to inspection checklist

DISPENSING
1. Present to patient in jewelry mat, not lab tray
2. Insure proper frame fit & patient satisfaction

OPTICIANU
OPTICIAN TRAINING

Lens Fabrication

The lens fabrication process can be divided into two major steps, surfacing and *finishing.* Understanding what takes place in each of these steps will help you to understand why certain jobs can be done "in house" and some sent off site. It will also help you foresee challenges lab technicians may face and help you communicate with them regarding these issues. Lab technicians are a wonderful source for information and are typically eager to speak with you about an order. They would much rather you speak with them at the time of placing an order than to have to call you after the fact which will delay the job and threaten customer satisfaction. The following infographic will provide you with a visual map of the lens fabrication process. This chapter will examine each of these steps in further detail.

Surfacing

Surfacing is the process by which a prescription is placed onto a lens and preparing its surface prior to being cut for the frame. Although large commercial ophthalmic labs do their own surfacing, this is not a process typically done at the small in-office lab. There are 4 steps involved in surfacing. These are 1) Blank selection 2) Generation 3) Polishing and Fining and 4) Hard coating.

Blank selection

A "blank" is a hockey puck size lens. There is no prescription within the "blank". The parameters preinstalled in the blank are only the front curvature (base curve), lens material such as polycarbonate, and the overall diameter.

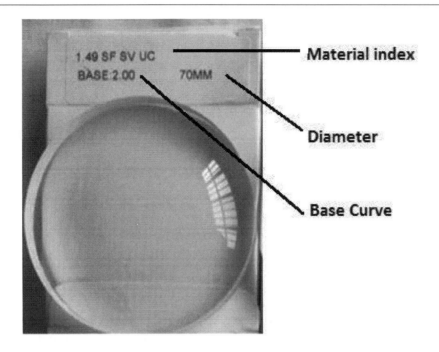

To know which blank to use for a given job, the lab technician inputs the patient's prescription and frame information into a computer program or uses a nomogram as seen below. Based on the nomogram, the lab technician is provided information about the lens blank to be used.   This will include such things as the base curve and blank size needed. The base curve does not affect the final prescription; however, it can affect the lens' ability to fit well within a frame. For example, an extremely wrapped frame will need a higher base curve in order to have the lens curve better match the frame curve. Similarly, a very flat frame will require a lower base curve lens.

The base curve may also affect off-axis clarity depending on the prescription ground into it. For these reasons, proper base curve selection is important both to ensure the lens will fit well in the fame and to ensure the best possible optical outcome.

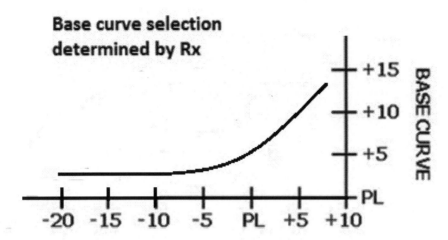

Base curve selection determined by Rx

Simplified graphical example of base curve selection criteria.
Notice how as prescription becomes more plus (+) in
power the necessary base curve increases.

Generating

Generation is the process by which the patient's prescription is ground into the back surface of the blank. The generator is a grinding instrument that etches the necessary curves into the back surface of the blank to achieve the desired prescription outcome.

In order to prepare the blank for prescription generation, there must be something fused to the blank to hold it in place in the generator. This is called a "block", and the process of adding the block to the blank is called "blocking".

In order to add the "block", the optical center of the blank must first be determined. The blank is placed in a lensometer and the location of the optical center is found. This is necessary in order to insure the lens is centered properly when the prescription is ground onto the lens. Tape is applied to the front surface of the lens to insure it does not become scratched during the blocking and generation process. The front surface of the blank (base curve) is not modified during the generation process.

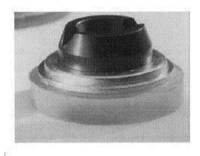

Lens blank with block applied and ready for generator

The blank is placed in a blocker which uses heated wax to fuse the block to the blank. Once the block is applied to the blank, it is placed in the generator which grinds the patient's prescription into the blank. Prescriptions are ground onto the **back** surface of the blank.

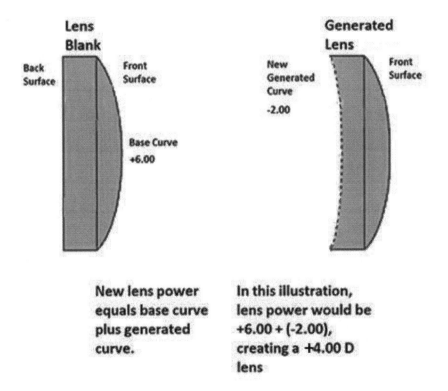

Lens Blank

Back Surface

Front Surface

Base Curve +6.00

Generated Lens

New Generated Curve -2.00

Front Surface

New lens power equals base curve plus generated curve.

In this illustration, lens power would be +6.00 + (-2.00), creating a +4.00 D lens

Fining and Polishing

When the lens is removed from the generator the back surface is rough, with a frosted appearance, from the process of grinding the prescription onto the blank. This multistep process is called "Fining and polishing". The process involves placing the lenses into a Finer which uses a polishing block called a lap. The first step in the finer involves the lens being polished by the lap in a circular motion against an abrasive fining pad similar to sandpaper to polish out the roughest parts created by the generator.

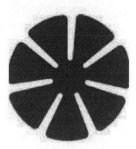

Typical fining pad

The second step uses a softer fining pad to remove further roughness. Step three polishes the lens again with an even softer fining pad and a polishing solution made of Aluminum oxide to create the crystal clear surface expected in the final product.

The block is detached and the protective tape applied prior to the process is removed by hand. When detaching the block, a small hammer is sometimes used, but if it can be done by twisting the lens, instead of a peeling motion of the block, there will be less chance of causing a lens defect.

Hard Coating

Once generated, scratch protection is applied to the lens. This process is called *Hard Coating*. The process of generating and polishing the prescription onto the back surface of the lens blank will leave the back surface of the lens soft and vulnerable to scratching. For this reason, a *hard coat* is applied to back side of the lens at this time.

A *hard coat* is a scratch protectant layer to prevent the newly generated lens from becoming scratched. The raw hard coat material is rather toxic, so must be handled with caution. Once applied to the lens, the hard coat solution is cured on to the surface of the lens using ultraviolet light to turn the liquid solution into a permanent hard scratch coating. Once cured, the coating is no longer toxic. And the lens can he safely handled.

Finishing

Finishing is the process of edging and mounting the surfaced lens blank for the selected frame. As opposed to surfacing, *finishing* is a process often done at in-office labs. The in-office lab will typically order a pre surfaced lens from a large commercial lab and *finish* it themselves. Finish includes 1) Edging 2) Mounting 3) Inspection and 4) Dispensing.

Edging

Now that the blank has the patient's prescription ground into its back surface and has been polished, it is time to cut the blank to fit the selected frame using an *Edger*. An edger is a lathe, using a diamond or ceramic grinding wheel, which cuts the blank to the shape of the frame. This process is called *"Edging"*.

The lab technician will use either a *pattern* (if provided by the optician or frame manufacturer) or a *tracer* to trace the frame shape directly. A *pattern* is a plastic disc the exact size and shape the lens needs to be in order to fit the frame. This is usually provided by the frame manufacturer to the optical shop that purchases the frame. If a pattern is not available, the lab technician places the frame into a *tracer*, a machine that traces the shape of the frame. The tracer then electronically sends the shape information to the edger to cut the lens into the appropriate shape.

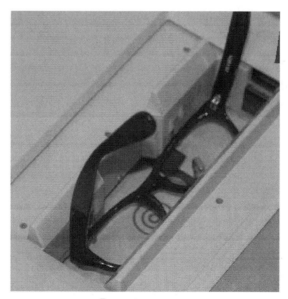

Frame tracer

Once the shape of lens needed is determined, the surfaced blank is prepped to be cut by the edger. Similar to the blocking step in lens generation, in edging the lens also must be blocked to give the edger a way to hold the lens securely while being cut. However, unlike the hot wax needed to hold the lens in a generator, the edging blocks are held in place by lightweight adhesive pads called *blocking pads*.

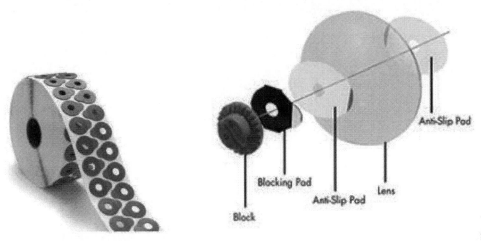

Roll of adhesive edging blocking pads.   Edger blocking pad and block mounting to lens.

Once mounted, the edger proceeds to cut the lens into the desired shape and cuts a groove or bevel in the edge depending on the frame design. Water is frequently pumped onto the lens by the edger to keep the lens from becoming to hot in the process. A hot lens is more prone to warpage, so a flow of water onto the lens is a standard feature of most edgers. Once complete, if the block can be removed using a gentle twisting motion of the lens instead of a peeling motion there will be less chance of creating a lens abrasion.

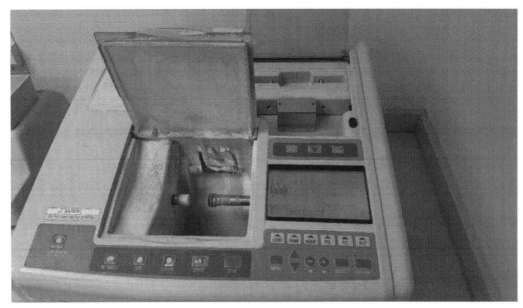

Typical in-office edger

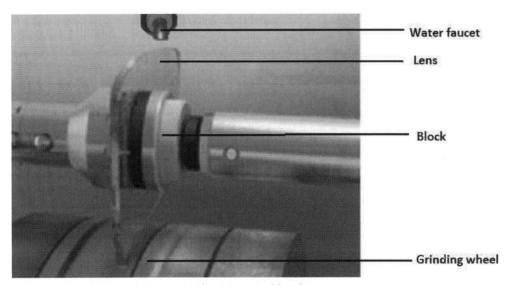

Lens mounted in edger.

The lens can be further ground or polished by a hand edger if needed for a perfect fit into the frame.

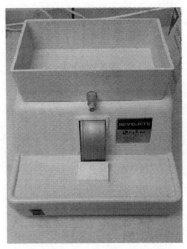

Example of manual hand edger.

Edging lenses can create toxic waste from the lens shavings and polishing compounds. These waste materials are funneled by the edger into bins stationed under the edger table. Edging high index materials will create a characteristically and strong odor, so your waste bin will need to be emptied frequently. Investing in a ventilation system for the lab is often a good idea for odor control.

Mounting

Mounting is the process of manually inserting the newly cut lens into the frame. Having a hand edger in the lab is useful for times when small modifications of the lens shape is needed to get a good fit in the frame.

Inspection

Once mounted, the completed job is inspected. An inspection looks to insure the optical center is in the proper placement, checking for scratches or other defects, and insuring there are no gaps between the frame and lens. An inspection checklist can be found on the following page.

Dispensing

The moment of dispense is the only moment the patient sees. All the hard work in the lab is for naught if a bad first impression is given at the moment the patient picks up their new glasses. The following pages give a checklist for dispensing a new pair of glasses.

Inspection & Dispensing Checklist

Inspection:

The following checks *must* be made on all glasses *just before they are given to the patient*:

_____ Power check

_____ Prism check

_____ Tint check

_____ Lens inspection for defects

_____ Frame inspection for defects

_____ Optical centers marked in lensometer

_____ Adjust frame

_____ Ensure optical center marks align with patient's PD (if dispensing PAL, must be checked on patient with template on lenses)

_____ Ensure bifocal line is appropriate height.

_____ Clean glasses

Dispensing:

Proper Eyeglass presentation and dispensing instruction:

_____ Proper eyeglass packaging.
Are they on a nice presentation mat with a quality eyeglass case?

_____ Exceed Expectations.
Include a cleaning spray bottle, cleaning cloth, or any other product or service.

_____ Provide clean and new-looking reading material for the patient's first look.
Is your reading material dog-eared and worn, or does it look crisp, new, and bright?

_____ Review all benefits of the glasses and premium upgrades.
By the time the patient picks up her glasses, she may have forgotten many of the benefits of the premium upgrades she purchased, such as an antireflective coating or a titanium frame. It is important to review these with her so when she goes home and hears a commercial for two pairs of glasses for $99, she does not feel buyer's remorse.

_____ Adjust the glasses, even if no adjustment is necessary.
Make the patient feel she is getting that customized fit.

_____ Compliment the patient on her new glasses.
Have you ever bought a nice piece of jewelry and the salesperson did not tell you how nice you looked in it? Probably not.

_____ Instruct patients on proper eyeglass care and handling.
1. Always store them in their case.
2. Never clean them with a paper product (Kleenex, paper towels, etc.), which can scratch the lenses. Use only a lint-free cleaning cloth.
3. Show proper cleaning with an eyeglass cleaner and silk cloth and recommend stores that sell them.

Troubleshooting problems at lens inspection

1. Lens haze:

Many times caused by the lens getting to hot. Plastic materials expand when heated, but antireflective coatings do not. So if the lens gets to hot during the edging process the stress caused to the AR coating by the expanding lens may cause the lens to appear hazy. If this is the case, ensure the edger is being properly cooled. It will likely have a water cooling system.

2. Linear scratches:

Scratches can occur at nearly any phase of lens creation. Protecting the lens is the best protection by the use of tape on the surface. Most lab supply stores sell surface protectant tape. By making sure the front surface (base curve) of a lens is taped while the back surface is being generated or making sure both sides are taped when being mounted in the frame or not being worked on, the lab can minimize the chance of scratches happening.

3. Circular scratches in center of lens:

Many times caused the lens being held to tightly in the edger. Modern edgers adjust the pressure based on the material being edged.   Excessive pressure and a permanent abrasion such as this is created, to little pressure and the lens slips and is edged incorrectly. Some materials are more prone to scratching, such as polycarbonate, so the edger will loosen its grip slightly. However, if the machine is told it is edging CR39 when it is really edging polycarbonate scratches may occur.

For softer materials, such as polycarbonate, some lab technicians will use two edging pads instead of one for added protection. If the lab technician ensures they have the edger set for the proper material and are using two pads, but the central scratches continue, the edger may need to be recalibrated by the edger's manufacturer technician.

4. Gaps between frame and lens:

This indicates the lens was edges a little too small. This could arise from a poor job of the tracer determining the size of the frame or possibly from the lens having to be manually edged prior to mounting to remove edge flaws from the automatic edger.

5. Rainbow appearance of the Antireflective coating:

This can be an indication that the lens is to large for the frame. Having to tighten the frame around a lens edged to large will cause the lens to warp. The aberrations caused by this warpage will appear as a rainbow or an oil slick on the antireflective coating. The lens may need to be removed from the frame and manually edges to slightly reduce its overall size.

6. Diffuse pinpoint scratches:

This is typically due to dust on the lens prior to application of the antireflective coating. Antireflective coatings are thinner than a grain of dust, so the dust will leave a button-hole within the coating. This will leave small areas on the lens without antireflective coating. These small areas, looking like a pinprick to the naked eye, is actually a spot on lens where a speck of dust prevented the antireflective coating from adhering.

7. Geographic blotching:

This is typically the antireflective coating not adhering to the lens. Although sometimes due to poor quality antireflective coatings, many times it is from the lens containing surface oils such as from fingerprints prior to the antireflective coating being applied.

Tinting tips and tricks

Different lens materials will absorb tints with variable rates of success. The material's polymer dictates how well or poorly a tint will penetrate. The following will help guide you towards both matching the best tint with lens material as well as be able to better educate your patients on how a given tint can be expected to perform on a given lens material.

Polycarbonate:

- The most difficult material to properly tint.
- Most tints use a carbon molecule that binds to a carbon molecule in plastic (CR-39) for its adhesion and stability. Polycarbonate chemical structure makes it resistant to this carbon binding.
- The best way to tint polycarbonate is to tint its scratch coating, however

historically the best scratch coats have been resistant to tinting.

- To overcome these limitations, manufacturing labs have recently developed scratch coats better able to absorb tints. However, in general, the best hard coat scratch protectors still make tinting polycarbonate more challenging than other materials.
- Always be sure the lens pairs being tinted are from the same manufacturer and same batch to insure consistent tinting.

Cr-39:

- Wider range of tinting color options and darkness levels than Polycarbonate due to its chemical make-up binding to tints more easily.
- Uncoated CR39 is the most porous of lens materials, making it easier to get a darker tint than other materials.
- Hard coated CR39 is still easier to tint than polycarbonate since the hard coat does not need to be as dense. This is due to CR39 being naturally less prone to scratching than Poly.

Trivex:

- Trivex is easy to tint, but since its material is not very porous the tint will not penetrate very deep. Therefore, harsh cleaners such as alcohol will fade the tint over time.
- Using a tintable hard coat may be the most stable method for tinting Trivex.

High Index:

- Able to be tinted well, however prepare for the process to take on the order of hours to complete. A tint that CR39 requires 10 minutes to complete may take a high index lens 3-4 hours to achieve the same outcome.

Rules for any material:

- Regardless of the material, lenses from different manufactures may tint differently depending on their processing and curing techniques. Even if from the same manufacturer, different batches of the same material may even tint slightly differently. So if replacing just one sunglass lens for a patient, be sure to educate them that the tint may not be a perfect match with the fellow lens. Replacing both lenses is typically the safer option to achieve the best cosmetic effect.

- Be sure to completely clean a lens using lens soap prior to tinting. Oils, dust, or other impurities will affect the uniformity of the tint.

- UV coating should be applied prior to any color tinting. This will prevent the tint color from fading.

- For lenses which you know have been previously hard or scratch coated, you will want to check with the lens manufacturer for their recommended tinting method. Some manufactures hard coatings will accept color and others will not, some manufacture coatings require a lower tint bath temperature or longer tint times. It is always our recommendation to check with the manufacturer first to avoid a tinting misadventure.

- All lens treatments such as tinting, UV treatments, and edge polishing must be done before an AR coat is applied. Tints should be made about 10% darker than intended prior to AR coating applications since the AR coating process will fade the tint by about 10%.

- For gradient tints, if you are experiencing a sharp demarcation between the lighter and darker areas instead of a smooth transition, your tint bath is likely to hot.

- In general, the hotter the tint bath the faster the lens will tint, however there are limits. Get the tint to hot and the color will decompose. Be sure to read the package insert for the color being used for recommended temperatures.

Tinting procedure:

Most in-office finishing labs will have a tint bath with 4-6 wells.

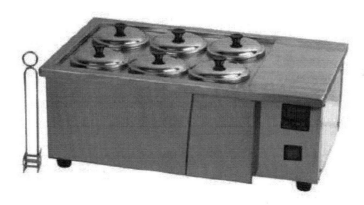

A typical tint bath with 6 wells.

Each tint bath well will contain a liquid dye created by mixing a Heat Transfer Fluid (usually not water) with a dye concentrate (or pill) and heated to 205° F. Using a Heat Transfer Fluid instead of water ensures the fluid within the bath heats quickly and is of a uniform temperature.

Although color concentrates or dye pills are available for nearly any color, your lab likely will not want to empty a tint bath to make room for a new color every time a new color is needed. Therefore, the tint bath wells will likely each contain one of the three primary colors… Blue, red, and yellow and maybe one for black given its popularity for tint color. From these colors alone almost any other color can be created using the following combinations.

Blue + Yellow = **Green**

Blue + Yellow + Red = **Black to Grey depending on concentration of colors**

Black + extra Red = **Yellowish Brown**

Yellowish Brown + extra red = **Natural Brown**

For more info on creating tints using only primary colors, visit http://optochemicals.com/tinting_colorguide.htm

Although tinting can be done manually, most labs use an electronic mechanical lever connected to a timer. The lever is mounted to the tint bath. It holds the lens and automatically dips the lens into the tint bath and raises it out of the bath based upon the timer setting. Darker tints will require longer tint times.

Chapter 9 test

1. The process by which a prescription is placed onto a lens is called what?
2. A "Blank" does not contain the final prescription. What 3 characteristics *does* it provide?
3. A plus power lens will generally have a steeper or flatter base curve when compared to a minus power lens?
4. The process by which the patient's prescription is ground into the blank is called what.
5. A lens with a base curve of +4.00 and a generated back curve power of -1.00 would have a prescription of what power?
6. When the lens is removed from the generator the back surface is rough from the process of grinding the prescription onto the surface. Removing this rough surface is called what?
7. Cutting the generated blank into a size that will fit into a frame is called what?
8. Areas of blotching in the Antireflective coating is often caused by what?
9. What is the most difficult lens material to get an even tint?

CHAPTER 10

Going from Good to Great

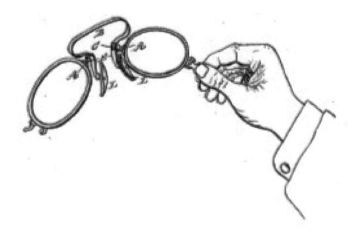

Moments of Truth

WHAT are Moments of Truth? Critical encounter points that shape patients' perception of their experiences. Critical encounter points are crucial moments of the buying experience that can make or break your impression with a patient. These can even be points at which you are not even present. The key is to think of all the points in time in which the patient may be forming an opinion of you and strive to make it a positive one.

For example, a classic Moment of Truth is when the patient walks through the door. Does the patient see a warm smile on your face and quick eye contact and a welcome (patient-centered), or does the patient see the staff behind the desk having personal conversations and acting oblivious that anyone has entered?

Now make your own list of *Moments of Truth* encounter points and list ideas on how to make each point a very patient-centered, positive experience. Discuss these with your optical manager. Afterwards, we will discuss a few you may not have thought of.

How many encounter points can you identify in your daily interactions?

1.

2.

3.

4.

5.

How can you turn each encounter point into a positive patient-oriented
   experience?

1.

2.

3.

4.

5.

There are many Moments of Truth you can come up with. Each office layout
may create a new supply of these encounter points and ways to make them
patient-centered. How many points did you come up with for which you, as an
optician, are not even present? These are tougher to think of but can be the most
important. There are two major Moments of Truth encounter points we must
prepare extra hard for since we will not be present to steer the outcome we want.
We must therefore lay the groundwork during the sale. These two moments are
when:

1. The patient sees an ad on TV for what appears to be a better deal than
   what he got from you.
2. When the patient's friend, neighbor, or family member talks about her
   own eyeglass-buying experience and new glasses.

Let's talk about No. 1 first. There is a common phenomenon in marketing
called *post-purchase dissonance*. In a nutshell, this is the post-purchase behavior of
consumers that drives them to seek out advertisements from your competitors to
reassure themselves that they did the right thing by buying from you and that they

got the best value. Keep in mind, all this happens *after* they have already bought from you! In order to get these patients' business again next year, we must be aware of this behavior and lay the groundwork during the sale to minimize the patients' post-purchase dissonance. There are a number of ways to do this.

1. As we discussed previously, talk to the patients about the benefits of all the lens and frame options they have included in their eyeglasses. This will have the patient leaving your office feeling good about their purchase and understanding the value of their purchase.

2. Give the patients itemized lists of all their lens and frame specifications. This way, when they see that ad for two pairs of glasses for $99, they will have a physical reminder that their own glasses (although they may have cost $400) were a much better value. Speak with your optical manager to see if your office has such a list for every patient. If not, suggest one be started and you will look like a genius!

The second Moment of Truth for which you will not be present is the most commonly feared marketing moment of any sales person: word-of-mouth advertising among friends and family. As an optician, the last thing you want is to have your patient's friend talk about how he got some great new "featherweight" lenses and have your patient wonder why you did not offer the same lenses to him! Don't have your patient learn something from a neighbor. Remember, *you* are the expert; that is *your* job!

To prevent this from happening, you must:

1. Educate your patients in multiple ways (verbal, with demos, and in writing after the sale) of all the benefits their eyeglasses provide. Your patient needs to become the community educator on eyeglass advancements and the one with bragging rights to owning the most advanced eyeglasses on the block! You do not want your patient learning anything from his neighbor; this will not be a positive Moment of Truth and will likely lead the patient to his neighbor's optician the next time he needs glasses.

2. Never prejudge your patient. By jumping to conclusions about your patient's ability to pay for an upgrade, you neglect to discuss lens options

that may be important to the patient and that he learns about from a neighbor.

3. Address the important concerns of every patient about their wants and needs connected to their new eyeglasses.

Opening Communication Channels

Many things in the life of an optician inhibit productive communication with the patient, the optician's single most important job. There is an old adage that "people don't care how much you know until they know how much you care." You must show each patient that he or she is the most important one of the day. The challenge is in doing this twenty or more times per day!

Additionally, communication done properly can be the best advertising for an optical center. Let us say that you sell a patient the best pair of glasses money can buy. The frames are made of titanium to help with the patient's allergies to other types of frame materials, the lenses are high-index and aspheric to help reduce the weight of the heavy prescription, and an antireflection coating was ordered to help the patient with symptoms of nighttime glare. Now suppose the patient is not made fully aware of the benefits of the purchase. The patient goes home with a large bill and feels resentment when he sees the next advertisement on TV touting two pairs of glasses for $99. He will think, "Wow, did I get taken!"

Now imagine the same patient encounter, but with extra time taken to ensure that the patient fully understood the *benefits* of what he purchased. Instead of paying $80 for an antireflective coat, he purchased "the state-of-the-art lens treatment to cut my nighttime glare problems!" Instead of paying for a high-index aspheric lens, he purchased "the most thin and lightweight lens available so my nose won't hurt anymore!" Speaking to the patient in terms of *benefits*, not optical lingo, will create a lifelong patient, one with armor to deflect any ads promoting cheaper glasses, and one who will speak to his neighbors about you.

The following are the most common obstacles to effective communication and how to overcome them.

> **Obstacle: Tech-talk**. This is speaking in our language, not the patient's. It's also speaking in terms of features, not benefits. A feature of an antireflective coating is its ten layers of silica precisely applied to create a reflection-free surface. Your patient typically will not care about this. A patient is concerned only about the benefit it provides: reducing his nighttime driving glare problem.
>
> Solutions:
> 1. Realize that we live in a different world from our patients. We must discuss benefits, not just features. In our patient's

world, "Antireflective coating" means nothing. "High index" or "aspheric" mean nothing. "PD, base curve, OC" mean nothing. When we speak *their* language, "antireflective coating" becomes the "less glare at night" coating. The "high index aspheric lens" becomes the "less weight on your nose" lens option.

2. Studies show that the best way to communicate a new term is to use the term first, then define it in terms of benefit. For example, "This problem you are having at night with glare, Mrs. Smith, I have just the solution. It is called an antireflective coating. It is specifically designed for people such as yourself who experience problems with glare from headlights. It makes nighttime driving much more comfortable."

Obstacle: Limited time. We have a limited amount of time to make the patient we are with feel like the most important patient of the day.

Solution:
1. Use of demos can explain a hundred words in a moment. Your office will likely have many wonderful demos of antireflective coatings and other lens options. Use them frequently!
2. Use the patient's name three times during ordering and pick-ups. There is no sound as sweet to your patient.

Obstacle: Waiting for the patient to make a complaint before offering a solution. Sometimes we feel as if telling patients about lens options makes us pushy salespeople. This feeling shortchanges the patients from very beneficial options that can completely change the way they feel about their glasses.

Solution:
1. Understand that *you* are the expert. This patient has come to you and trusted his eye care to you for a reason. He feels *you* will provide the best care. So provide it—let him know all of the latest and greatest in lens options.
2. Do not wait for the patient to ask about a "better lens" before

explaining AR coats, high index, or photochromatics. The last thing we want is for the patient's neighbor to be the first to tell *our* patient of a lens option he would have benefited from.

3. Ask lifestyle questions to introduce lens options. Ask the patient if his high prescriptions seem heavy. If so, discuss high-index and aspheric lenses. Ask the patient if he ever notices glare at nighttime or on the computer. If so, discuss antireflective coatings. The patients will appreciate the interest you take in their well-being!

Obstacle: Prejudging a patient's ability to afford a given lens option. It is human nature to want to pigeonhole your patients into financial categories based on their insurance, appearance, or a host of other factors. This obstacle will shortchange the patients from receiving the best pair of glasses to meet their needs.

Solution:

Remember, everyone deserves the best, or at least the *opportunity* to receive the best. Never assume someone cannot or will not pay for a lens option that is truly the best for the patient. Let the patients be the ones to inform you what they can or cannot afford.

Obstacle: Filtered listening. Filtered listening is anytime either you or the patient listen with a preconceived notion about what is being said. For example, you may say, "I see the doctor has you starting in bifocals for the first time," and the patient may reply with, "What! You think I'm old now, too!" This is because patients often associate the word "bifocal" with "old." In another example, the patient says, "I am on a budget, so I only want what I really need." And you may hear, "I want the cheapest pair of glasses you have." This is because you associate the word "budget" with "tight-wad". One person's budget is not another person's budget. This person deserves the same attention to lifestyle prescribing as anyone. Besides, he may consider lens option upgrades as something that falls in the category of "something he really needs," especially if he has lived a life complaining of heavy glasses or glare.

Solution:

1. Clean the filter. Really listen to what is being said as well as what you are saying, and try to avoid making assumptions.

2. Ask patients if they have any questions. This will open the lines of communication and help declog any wrong perceptions trapped in the filter.

3. Have the patient repeat back to you what you have said. This will ensure the patient fully understands why they would benefit from a given lens option.

Obstacle: Body language. Yes, your body itself can become an obstacle to efficient communication.

Solution:

1. See yourself from an out-of-body experience. Are you writing in the chart while talking to the patient? Are you making eye contact or watching other patients during your discussion? Are you chewing gum or playing with your hair? None of these will exactly open up the lines of communication.

2. Lean in slightly toward the patient.

3. Make eye contact.

4. Open your posture. Avoid crossed arms or legs.

Starting (and ending) the Conversation

So here you are, thrown to the wolves, and you see a patient walking toward the door. Your heartbeat quickens, your palms become sweaty, and you forget your own name or how you even landed yourself in this position. Hopefully, you are a new optician and not a seasoned one experiencing this!

Sweat not; the following map will help give you the confidence to navigate through your first patient encounter. The following is only a general outline. As you gain confidence, you will likely discover your own additions to include on the map and make it your own. But for now, you need to know where you are, where you are going, and how you are going to get there.

Let's return to the plight of our new optician seeing his first patient walking toward him. Our optician remembers his map and proceeds as follows.

1. **Greet** the patient! This sounds simplistic, but it is often forgotten. Welcome the patient to your optical center and introduce yourself *by name*. For example, "Welcome! My name is Susan and I will be your optician today." Many great optical consultants will recommend not using the word *optician* since many patients are not clear on what it is. They often confuse that job title with optometrist, ophthalmologist, or even the lab technician. Other titles you can use in its place are "frame stylist," "fashion consultant," or "eyewear specialist". Speak with your manager about what the proper usage of your job title should be.

2. **Ask** "What can I help you with today?" Asking an open-ended question such as this will get the conversation and eyeglass selection process headed in the right direction on our map. Follow up by asking patients to be as specific as they can about the problems they are having or the goal they are hoping to achieve.

3. **Show** a demonstration of solutions to their problems. Your optical department will likely have demonstrations of everything from antireflective lenses to the difference in thickness between high-index lenses and conventional plastic lenses.

4. **Recommend.** This is the step in which you show your true professional knowledge. The worst thing you can say is, "Do you want … ?" You are

the professional. Say, "I recommend … on your glasses to solve your complaint of …" For example, for a person who told you he wanted lighter-weight lenses, this recommendation step would sound like this: "Mrs. Smith, you stated that you wanted to have lighter-weight lenses in your glasses. I would recommend you get a high-index aspheric lens. This lens is made up of the thinnest and lightest material available. If we pair this lens with a titanium frame, we will truly have the lightest pair of glasses possible."

5. ***Present price.*** Presenting the final price to a patient is often the most difficult stage for a new optician. You add everything up and arrive at a total of six hundred dollars, and your first thought is, "Oh my! I would never spend this much on glasses. How can I ask this patient to?" The difference is two-fold. 1) You are not your patient. Maybe your patient just spent $2,000 on a new wardrobe and $200 on a haircut. Investing $600 on a new pair of glasses may seem like a bargain. 2) You may be a very healthy individual with a light prescription. Without knowing what it is like to have to wear a very thick prescription or have to put up with glare from your cataracts, it is difficult to place a value on a premium pair of glasses with high index lenses and an antireflective coating. Remember, the patients always deserve the best. As long as you are meeting their needs, you have no reason to feel guilty about the price. If the patient says that the glasses cost too much, ask the patient which benefit he is willing to give up in order to bring the price down. Your job is to offer a product to meet the patient's needs; it is up to the patient to decide what he can and cannot afford and what benefits he can live without. Present the price with confidence and without prejudice as to what you think the patient can afford to pay.

6. ***Collect.*** Every office will have different collection policies, but in general it is best to collect the entire purchase price before the patient leaves the office. There will always be the patients who ask if they can simply make a deposit. Speak with your office manager about these cases. When collecting the money, it is best to simply state the total price of the purchase and ask if the patient will be paying by cash, check, or credit card; then be quiet and let the patient respond. It is at this collection

step that many opticians feel guilty over the price, which prompts them to ask the patient if he would rather just put a deposit down. *Avoid this temptation.* What other business do you know that allows you to place an order for a customized product but not pay for it in full? Yet somehow, this has become a standard practice in the optical world and seriously affects the offices' cash flow. Just because you do not make the patient pay up-front does not mean your office will not have to pay for the materials up-front. So do your office a favor and expect full payment when glasses are ordered.

Defusing a Dissatisfied Patient

A recent study showed that premium car buyers who had to take their new car back to the dealer for repair work and were treated respectfully during the process had a greater overall satisfaction with their car than owners of the same type of car who never had to take the car back to the dealer for repairs. This shows us that when patients returns to us with a problem with their new glasses, we should see this as an opportunity, a Moment of Truth, in which we can make the patient more loyal to us than if they had never had a problem in the first place.

The following is designed to help you communicate more efficiently with patients who may not, let's say, be in the happiest of moods. In any retail setting, you are bound to run across patients who, either rightly or wrongly, have a grudge to bear against you, your company, or life in general. You are the one they are intent on taking it out on.

The primary reason dissatisfied patients seem to be on the offensive from the beginning is that they fear we will trivialize their complaint. Turn the tables and be *more* gracious than the day you sold them the glasses. Here are steps to quickly turn a dissatisfied patient encounter into a pleasant exchange. Do not be afraid to apologize during any of these steps if you discover you or a coworker made a mistake in the fabrication of the patient's eyeglasses. An apology can go a long way in building rapport.

1. **Introduce yourself** and state that *you* will be the one to solve the problem. This is not to say you may not need to rely on others for guidance, but you are the patient's point person and will see that a resolution to the problem occurs.

2. **Thank the patient** for coming back to let us solve his problem. This will help the patient drop his guard. He is expecting a fight, or at least a trivialization of his complaint. A simple "Thank you for bringing this to my attention" will smooth the road to finding a solution for both you and the patient.

3. **Listen.** Let the patient vent, then ask detailed questions using FOLDAR to get a clearer understanding of the problem. FOLDAR is an acronym for the questions you need to ask to get to the root of the problem.

FOLDAR stands for:

F: Frequency. How often does the problem occur? All day or just at
   certain times of the day?

O: Onset. When did the problem first occur? When you first put on the
   glasses, or has it started more recently?

L: Location. Where is the problem? One eye or both eyes?

D: Duration. How long does the problem last?

A: Associated symptoms. Are there any other symptoms accompanying the
   one you are describing?

R: Relief. Does doing anything help the symptoms? Such as closing one
   eye or taking the glasses off?

The venting is for the patient's benefit; FOLDAR is for yours.

4. **Show you understand** how the patient feels. Say "You feel _____
   because _____." For example, say to the patient "**You feel
   frustrated because** that right eye of yours just isn't seeing up to either
   of our expectations." This may seem corny, but it works wonders. It also
   works when a patient unloads his life's troubles on you. It shows the
   patient you are not an adversary and that you understand why the patient
   is back in your office.

5. **Solve the problem**.

6. Thank the patient. Yes, thank the patient again for coming back so we
   could solve his problems. He is doing us a favor; he is not an annoyance
   in our day. By coming back to vent with us and allow us to solve his
   problem, he is not venting with a neighbor!

Get Off Our Buts!

Patients are interested in solutions to their problems, not excuses. It is common to reply to a patient's request with "I would, but …" or "I wish I could, but …." Excuses contain "but …"; solutions contain "what I can do is …." Remember, *patients do not enter our offices with problems, only solutions waiting to be discovered!*

Are we doing all we can to create solutions and not excuses?

For each of the following situations, think about an excuse, something that contains the word "but." Then think of a solution. *Solve the problem! Make it happen!* There are no single correct answers. Discuss them with your optical manager to make sure that your solution is actually possible. The goal here is to make you feel empowered in your job and to think with a patient-centered mindset.

Situations:

1. Patient calls one week after ordering to see if glasses are ready. Glasses are not ready yet.

   Excuse:

   Solution:

2. Patient is upset with us that insurance authorization is not in yet. We have been calling for a week to get the authorization, but the insurance company is dragging its feet.

   Excuse:

   Solution:

3. During a busy day, we forget to call a cab for a patient. Patient has been waiting for an hour and is obviously upset.

   Excuse:

   Solution:

4. Patient wants to replace a broken frame that is now discontinued.

    Excuse:

    Solution:

Features vs. Benefits

Patients do not buy *features*, they buy *benefits*. What is the difference? Features are inherent properties of a material or product. For example, features of polycarbonate lenses are its light weight, UV protection, and thinness. Do patients actually care about any of these things? Actually, no! So why would they pay extra for polycarbonate lenses? Because of the *benefits* these things provide. What benefit does a lightweight lens give? More comfort. What benefit does UV protection provide? Better eye health. What benefit does a thin lens provide? A more cosmetically appealing pair of glasses.

When selling glasses, it is essential to describe the benefits of lens options, not just the features. For each of the following examples, list the features and the benefits of each feature. Discuss this with your team leader or manager for ideas on how to present each lens option through demonstrations your office may have.

1. Antireflective coating

     Features   Benefits

2. Titanium frame

     Features   Benefits

3. Sunglasses

     Features   Benefits

4. High Index lenses

     Features   Benefits

5. Aspheric lenses

     Features   Benefits

Dispensing Checklist

The time of dispensing glasses should be considered one of our Moments of Truth. This is one of those make-or-break moments when a patient will form a lasting impression of the service you provide. There are two parts of dispensing eyeglasses that must be kept in mind. One is the *Nuts and Bolts* and the other is the *Warm and Fuzzies*. The *Nuts and Bolts* deal with insuring the proper power and fit of the glasses on the patient. The *Warm and Fuzzies* deal with making the patient feel as if he is receiving the most important pair of glasses you have ever handled. Recall the phrase we learned earlier: *The patient doesn't care how much you know* (the nuts and bolts) *until they know how much you care* (the warm and fuzzies). This means you can create the most accurate pair of glasses known to man, but if you just give them to the patient with no regard for the patient's emotional interest in the glasses, the patient will likely find fault with them. We will now discuss the *Nuts and Bolts* and *Warm and Fuzzies* to make you look like a genius optician.

The Nuts and Bolts

The following checks *must* be made on all glasses *just before they are given to the patient*. There is nothing more embarrassing than having a patient return unhappy with her glasses when one of these basic checks have not been made. These checks, when performed in the order listed below, will help you ensure the proper fit and function of the glasses *before* the patient notices a problem. It may be a good idea to make a copy of these checks and have them posted in your dispensing area as a reminder.

_____ Power check

_____ Prism check

_____ Tint check

_____ Lens inspection for defects

_____ Frame inspection for defects

_____ Optical centers marked in lensometer

_____ Adjust frame

_____ Ensure optical center marks align with patient's PD
(if dispensing PAL, must be checked on patient with
template on lenses)

_____ Ensure bifocal line is appropriate height.

_____ Clean glasses

The Warm and Fuzzies

Now that we have a pair of glasses that will knock the socks off the patient, how do we present them in a way that will make the patient feel it is the most important pair of glasses you have ever dispensed? Simple; just remember the following.

1. Proper eyeglass packaging.
   How do you package the eyeglasses when you deliver them to the patient? Are they in a dirty plastic tray or are they on a nice presentation mat with a quality eyeglass case?

2. Exceed Expectations.
   Do you provide anything not otherwise expected by the patient? Every patient expects a clean pair of glasses, so simply having them spotless isn't enough. If it's OK with your optical manager, include a cleaning spray bottle, cleaning cloth, or any other product or service that will make the patient feel as if she is getting more than she paid for.

3. Provide clean and new-looking reading material for the patient's first look through the new glasses.
   When dispensing glasses, you will likely want to have the patient try to read something so you can ensure the prescription is correct. Is your reading material dog-eared and worn, or does it look crisp, new, and bright?

4. Handle glasses like jewelry.
   Whether you are dispensing a $900 pair of glasses or a $100 pair, the

patient has a lot invested in the glasses, and receiving them is a major moment for the patient. Treat the glasses like the jewelry that they are. Hold them gingerly and speak of them fondly.

5. Review all benefits of the glasses and premium upgrades.
    By the time the patient picks up her glasses, she may have forgotten many of the benefits of the premium upgrades she purchased, such as an antireflective coating or a titanium frame. It is important to review these with her so when she goes home and hears a commercial for two pairs of glasses for $99, she does not feel buyer's remorse for the amount she spent in your office. Additionally, a well-informed patient becomes a spokesperson for you to all of her friends and neighbors. We always want our patients to educate their friends about the best lens options, not to have our patients *be educated* by a friend about a lens option they should have received. Patients *do* talk about their glasses; make sure your patient is fully aware of all the premium benefits of her glasses.

6. Adjust the glasses, even if no adjustment is necessary.
    Patients want to feel as if their glasses are custom fit; part of this includes your making adjustments. Even if the frame fits perfectly on the patient, do some slight fiddling with the frame to make the patient feel she is getting that customized fit.

7. Compliment the patient on her new glasses.
    Have you ever bought a nice piece of jewelry and the salesperson did *not* tell you how nice you looked in it? Probably not. Do the same with your patients after you give them their glasses, and the patients will think fondly of you when they think fondly of their new glasses.

8. Instruct patients on proper eyeglass care and handling.
    Just as you would never buy jewelry without being taught how to care for it, you should never have patients leave your office without teaching them how to care for their glasses:

    1. Always store them in their case.
    2. Never clean them with a paper product (Kleenex, paper towels,

etc.), which can scratch the lenses. Use only a lint-free cleaning cloth.

3. Always put them on and remove them by holding both temples to avoid getting them out of adjustment.

4. Show proper cleaning with an eyeglass cleaner and silk cloth and recommend stores that sell them.

Cover Your Bases for Accurate Ordering

Have you ever had that nagging feeling that something just has not been done that you really needed to do? Well, hopefully if you remember the steps for ordering a pair of glasses, this feeling will never again happen to you (at least not at work!) The following are the steps that must occur, in order, to get you from the batter's box, across all the bases, and back to home plate for each glasses order. There is no jumping from first base to third base in baseball or in preparing your order.

> First Base: To get to first, **make sure you have a current copy of the patient's prescription, recognize if it is in (+) or (–) cylinder form, and record this on the order form.** It is amazing how often an optician will spend a half hour with a patient selecting a frame only to find out the patient expected the optician to be psychic and know what their prescription is. Get a copy in your hands before the selection process begins. This also will help you make better recommendations on the type of frame and lens that would work best for the patient's prescription. Make sure to double-check the prescription you record for accuracy.

> Second Base: To get to second base, **properly adjust the selected frame**. This must occur prior to any measurements. If, for example, the frame is not adjusted until after a seg height is measured, your adjustment would change the final location of the seg height to something other than what you intended. Congratulations, you are now in scoring position!

> Third Base: Getting to third requires **measuring the patient's PD**. No pair of glasses can accurately be fabricated by the laboratory without this.

> Home Plate: To get across home plate, **measure for the seg height,** if one is needed.

There are several additional things to keep in mind that can minimize errors in completing your order.

1. Always use three decimal places when writing prescriptions. For example, a power of +2.50 should not be abbreviated to +2.5, nor should a power

of -3.00 be abbreviated to -3. The same rule applies to the axis. A two-digit axis, such as an axis of 10, should be recorded as 010.

2. Do not use a degree sign (°) after the axis when placing your order. This can sometimes be mistaken for a zero (0), and the lab might fabricate the lens with an incorrect axis.

3. If only one lens in the patient's glasses is being replaced, be sure to measure the base curve of the fellow lens and specify that the new lens be made with the same base curve. Having both lenses with the same base curve will help ease the patients' adaptation to their new glasses.

4. If the prescription calls for only a spherical lens with no cylinder component, always write DS (for diopter sphere) or just Sphere after the spherical power. This lets the reader know that you did not simply forget to complete writing the prescription's cylinder component.

Recommend, and the Selling Part is Done for You (Increasing your second pair and average dollar sales)

"Do you want …" is a phrase used by novice salespeople. There is no expertise or knowledge of the patient reflected in such a statement.

"I recommend, based on what you've been telling me, that we go with … " shows expertise, professionalism, and a true knowledge of the patient's wants and needs. It is not based on preconceived notions of a person's ability to pay, but rather respects the patients enough to recommend the best solutions to their problems.

The only way you can get to the point of making recommendations is to ask open-ended questions to get to know the patient's wants and needs. The difference between an open-ended question and a closed-ended question is the amount of information gleaned from the answer. For example, a common closed-ended question for a novice optician to start a conversation is, "Are you looking for a pair of glasses similar to what you have now?" Aside from the fact that the whole reason the patient came in to see us is that they have an unmet need, an even bigger issue is, what are you going to do with the answer? What if the patient says no? You haven't gotten any information about what it is they want to change about their glasses. What if the patient says yes? You may then assume that they are talking about the shape, when in fact they are talking about the weight!

A better question would be an open-ended one that allows the patient to elaborate on the topic. In this case, the question may be worded, "What about your glasses do you like?" or, "What about your current glasses don't you like?" This will enable you to gather much more useful information that you can then package as a recommendation.

Examples of opened-ended questions:

1. What do you like about your current glasses?
2. What don't you like about your current glasses?
3. Where do you find your vision most troublesome? (to glean interest in add-ons)
4. What do you do for a living? (to glean interest in second pairs, add-ons)
5. How may I help you? (After telling the patient your name!)
6. What do you currently use for sunglasses? (increase second pairs)
7. What kind of leisure activities are you involved in? (increase second pairs)

8. Are you looking for any particular type of frame?

9. What do you want your frames to say about you? (increase second pairs)

10. What type of activities are you involved in outside work? (increase second pairs)

When making your recommendations, make sure to reference what the patient has told you when you arrive at your recommendations, and be sure to start with the phrase "Based upon what you have told me, I would recommend …." The patient is there to get your expert opinion, so give it!

There is another benefit of this recommend-based philosophy to patient interaction; it improves your average dollar sale without you having to feel like a pushy salesperson, and the patient feels better served. This is because you are starting with a top-down approach, as opposed to a bottom-up approach, at creating a pair of glasses. For example, let's say a patient walks up to you with a prescription for his new glasses. Instead of getting to know the patient through open-ended questions, you simply say, "Do you want a titanium frame to make them lighter weight?" Your next question is, "Do you want a high index lens?" followed by "Do you want an aspheric lens?" and "Do you want an AR coat to help with the glare?" This is a bottom-up approach. You are starting with nothing, and bit by bit piecing together a pair of glasses for your patient. This is excruciatingly painful for the patient, as he sees the bill getting higher and higher, and painful for you as well as you wait for his answers. When you are done, the patient is looking a huge bill and not understanding how it all happened.

By contrast, let us say that through your open-ended questions that you find the patient's chief goal for getting new glasses is to make the -5.00 prescription more comfortable to wear and look cosmetically better. You then say, *"Based upon what you have been telling me, I recommend we go with a titanium frame matched with a high-index aspheric lens. This will provide you with the ultimate in a thin and lightweight pair of glasses. Additionally, I recommend we put an antireflective treatment on the lenses, since this coating will not only provide additional visual comfort by allowing greater light transmission through your higher prescription and reducing glare, but will also make your lenses seem invisible to anyone looking at you, which you said was important to you as well."*

This is an example of a top-down approach. You are presenting the patient with a package that meets his needs. No more and no less. The patient also understands why you are making the recommendations, since they are completely based on his own answers to your questions. Let's say the bill now comes to $500, and the patient flinches. This is fine, because we have started with what the patient needs based on his own goals. There has been no hard selling, so the patient has no hard feelings toward you about the price. The patient knows he is the one who brought the two of you to this point and why. Let him now be the one to prioritize his goals to get a pair of glasses within his budget. How do we do this? Simply by asking, *"Based upon your goals of a thin and lightweight pair of glasses that are also cosmetically appealing, which goals are most important to you, and which ones can you do without?"*

More often than not, if the patient can afford it, he will follow your recommendations. You have educated him, and he sees the value of the premium package in meeting his goals. Sometimes, however, the patient can afford only a basic frame with a basic plastic lens. At least the patient knows that you, unlike any other optician, took the time to get to know his needs, and so next year he will come back to you for those lightweight glare-free lenses the two of you discussed.

For each of the following patients, provide an example of a novice sales job and an example showcasing your true expertise and professionalism.

1. A child (who always needs polycarbonate) who plays soccer.
2. A person whose prescription is a +4.00 DS OU and wants thinner, lighter lenses.
3. A person in sales who makes presentations in front of large audiences and wants to look her best.
4. An elderly person who has red marks on his nose from the weight of his frame.
5. A middle-aged person with a deep tan.
6. A contact-lens wearer.
7. A person who complains of nighttime glare interfering with his driving.

Troubleshooting

What do you do when a patient comes into your office saying she does not see well with her new glasses? This will be a frequent part of your job, occurring often, so this is not a topic to be taken lightly. Your job is to do all you can to find the source of the problem before sending the patient back to the doctor for an Rx re-check. This scenario is embarrassing for the patient and time-consuming for the doctor. There are times when it is necessary, but the better goalie you can be in preventing unnecessary doctor visits for Rx checks, the happier both the doctor and the patient will be.

Patients' complaints that they are not seeing well through their new glasses may arise from one or several sources:

1. **Prescription error:** The doctor arrived at an incorrect prescription for the patient.
2. **Lab error:** The lab made an error in lens fabrication that was not caught.
3. **Optician error:** The ordering optician made incorrect measurements, incorrect assumptions, or made transposing errors from the doctor's prescription.
4. **Patient perception error:** The patients either have an incorrect perception about their visual potential or about how long it may take to become adjusted to their new glasses prescription.
5. **A visual/perceptual problem:** New prescriptions may not always permit adaptation, regardless of the amount of time given to wearing the new glasses, if there is too large of a change from the patient's previous glasses.

Let us discuss each one in more detail.

Prescription error

Do doctors make errors? Sometimes. The doctor uses many sources of information when arriving at a prescription for a patient. The primary source is from the *subjective refraction.* This is the infamous "What is better, 1 or 2" test. What is maddening for doctors about this test is the very *subjective* nature of it; the doctor cannot see what the patients are seeing and tell them which choice to make. The patients must decide for themselves. Doctors much prefer cut-and-dry, *objective*, decision making.

Doctor: "Where does it hurt?"
Patient: "My toe."
Doctor: "This one?"
Patient: "Ouch!"
Doctor: "OK then, let's do an X-ray of it."
Doctor: "Hey, look here! It's broken; see the crack in your bone? This is proof it's broken and explains your pain. Let me wrap it and get you a prescription for a pain killer."

This is the type of conversation doctors like to have. It is very *objective*, meaning evidence-based. In comparison, here is a typical conversation that leads a doctor to write a prescription for glasses:

Doctor: I am going to show you a series of two lenses; you tell me which one makes the letters *more* clear. OK?
Patient: OK.
Doctor: This is lens number one … or lens number two?
Patient: They are both kinda blurry.
Doctor: Again, just tell me which one is *more* clear. Lens number one … or two?
Patient: Two. I guess.
Doctor: Please don't guess. If they both look the same, it is OK to say they look the same. Let's look at the next two lenses now. This is number three … or four?
Patient: That number two was better than either of these!
Doctor: We have moved beyond those. Again, which lens is *more* clear?
Patient: Well, number four is, if I have to guess!

This illustrates the *subjective* nature of arriving at a glasses prescription. Accurate patient feedback is essential at arriving at a good endpoint. Fortunately for the doctor, he or she is able to rely on additional sources of information. These other sources include:

1. The patient's current prescription.
2. Any complaints the patient is having about his current glasses.
3. Any medical conditions that may adversely alter the patient's responses.
4. The confidence the doctor has in the patient's responses.

For example, if a patient has no complaints with his current glasses, but the doctor finds a large change in their prescription, the doctor is not likely to prescribe the entire change even if it significantly improves the patient's vision. Another example of a scenario that happens frequently is in a patient with cataracts. Cataracts will cause a patient to enter the doctor's office with a complaint of decreased vision. During the subjective refraction, the patient will usually like additional minus-power added to their prescription. Often this can lead to a significant improvement in their tested visual acuity in the exam room. Unfortunately for the patient, if the doctor prescribes this cataract-induced minus-power shift, the patient will complain of eyestrain. It is therefore up to the doctor to realize that the power change is caused by the cataracts and know that, for whatever the reason, cataract patients do not respond well to new glasses with this change.

Lab error

Do labs make errors? Sometimes. Labs are busy places where lenses are made quickly by a machine. However, wherever there are machines, there is always the human element. Lab technicians must input data into the equipment and check the work that is completed. Data can be missed and flawed lenses can be passed.

Optician error

Do opticians make errors? Despite the best efforts of this book, sometimes. Optician errors can arise from any number of situations: erroneous PD measurements; incorrectly assuming the patient wanted a trifocal when they wanted a bifocal; transposition errors when copying the doctor's prescription; or not matching the best progressive lens design for the patient's lifestyle.

Patient perception error

Do patients make mistakes? Sometimes, but we can never let them know it. What we can do, though, is make them aware of what may be causing their erroneous perceptions. For a new prescription that has had anything but a very mild change, reassure patients that it may take a week to get completely used to their new glasses. Always review the patients' chart to be sure there aren't cataracts or macular degeneration that the patients have forgotten about, which may explain the patients feeling as if their glasses still don't help them see well. Patients often have an erroneous perception of their visual potential.

Visual-perception problem

Do the glasses themselves, even if the prescription is correct, cause problems? Sometimes. These are called visual-perception problems. These are the problems created by a different image size or shape projected onto the retina than was projected by the previous glasses, even if the new image is clearer. A large change in the prescription's sphere power will cause a change in image size and a large change in a prescription's cylinder correction will change the image shape. Examples of visual-perception problems include the following:

The tilted table problem: Patients may complain that a flat surface, like a table, looks tilted. What does this mean? If the flat surface is tilted right/left, then this is likely an astigmatism change. Recall that with astigmatism, one axis has a different power than the axis 90 degrees away. This creates varying magnifications around the lens from 1–180°. If this magnification is different from the previous glasses, the brain will take a step back and wonder what is wrong. As long as there has not been too large of a change, the brain will usually adapt over time.

What if the table is perceived as tilted toward or away from the patient? This is usually a result of a change in the vertex distance, base curve, or pantoscopic tilt from their previous glasses. This is harder for the brain to adapt to since it is not the actual prescription causing the magnification difference, but rather a lens (external factor)-induced magnification difference. Finding a difference in one of these parameters from their previous glasses is likely the only way to solve the patients' symptoms.

Fortunately, at the end of this chapter is a Troubleshooting Analysis Form that will help you do just that.

Wow, that's big! (Or small): Patients may complain that images appear bigger or smaller through their new glasses. Prescription changes that add plus power will likely yield images appearing larger than they should be. The additional plus power projects a more magnified image onto the retina than their previous glasses did. This is usually solved simply by having the patient continue wearing the lenses for a week. An easy way to help the patient adapt is to say, "Through your previous glasses, images were perceived as being smaller than they really were; now with the new glasses, images are the correct size, but the brain is seeing them as relatively larger. It may take a week, but the brain will adapt." It is best to place the adaptation blame onto some third party, like the brain, so the patient does not feel we are placing the blame directly on them!

A change in prescription that adds more minus-power will cause the opposite effect; images may seem slightly smaller than with the patient's old glasses. Like before, as long as the prescription is correct, the patient will adapt within about a week.

As you can see, most of these errors are just from people being people. People make mistakes. Taking care in checking your work will help, but people still make mistakes. This book cannot keep those from happening, but it can help you navigate the waters when you find the source of the patient's problems. How? The next page is the Troubleshooting Analysis Worksheet. Use it on all of your patients who have any complaints about their new glasses before sending them back to the doctor for an Rx re-check. Tear it out and make copies for yourself and your coworkers.

Not all fabrication errors require a remake of the glasses. *ANSI standards* specify how much off-prescription a lens can be and still be acceptable. ANSI standards are developed by a private, nonprofit organization that develops norms and guidelines for a wide range of industry-grade products, including prescription glasses. You will want to obtain a copy of these standards and post it where you perform your glasses analysis. A copy of these standards can be obtained at www. ansi.org. ANSI standards typically allow less than a 0.25D difference for low powers and less than a 2-percent difference in high powers. So these standards pretty much require the glasses to be spot-on to the prescription.

Here is a key for a few of the abbreviations on the Troubleshooting Worksheet:

Pano: The pantoscopic tilt. Recall that this is the angle the lenses make with the face. This should be about 10 degrees.

OC: The optical centers. This should be directly over the pupils. Recall the way to find the optical centers is to place the lens in a lensometer, center the mires, and use the ink marker in the lensometer to identify the location.

Seg Ht: This is the seg height—how high the bifocal is on the frame.

DBOC: The distance between the optical centers.

DBS: The distance between the bifocal segments.

Patient's PD. The distance between the patient's pupils, as measured with a pupilometer or PD ruler. Recall that this should be the same as the distance between optical centers in most cases.

Troubleshooting Analysis Worksheet

Patient Name:_____   Date:_____

Chief complaint:_____

_____

Wearing time: _____

Prior glasses

Material:_____ Base Curve Horiz OD_____ OS_____   <u>Check if OK</u>
                                         Vert OD_____ OS_____   Pano [ ]   OC [ ]
Lens Style:_____   Vertex dist [ ]

	Sphere	Cyl	Axis	Prism
Rx OD					Seg Ht _____
OS					Seg Ht _____
Add +			DBOC _____	DBS _____

Prescribed Rx

	Sphere	Cyl	Axis	Prism
Rx OD				
OS				
Add +			Patient's PD _____	

New Glasses

Material:_____ Base Curve Horiz OD_____ OS_____   <u>Check if OK</u>
                                         Vert OD_____ OS_____   Pano [ ]   OC [ ]
Lens Style:_____   Vertex dist [ ]

	Sphere	Cyl	Axis	Prism
Rx OD					Seg Ht _____
OS					Seg Ht _____
Add +			DBOC _____	DBS _____

Suggested action _____

Keeping Track of Your Patients

Have you ever placed an order for a product and felt as if the salesperson suddenly gave up caring about you or tracking your order as soon as you walked out the door. Of course you have. You realize the salesperson does not have as much vested interest in the order as you do, but still you wish he would at least act like he does. As an optician, we need to keep patients from thinking this of you.

Your patients will be spending hundreds of dollars on a product you sell them and will hear every word you tell them regarding when they can expect to receive their glasses. Your patients will be sitting by the phone the day you promised the glasses would be ready and fuming if the phone is not ringing.

Your goal: Call the patient BEFORE the patient calls you.

Keeping your patients regularly updated on the status of their order will go a long way in taking you from being a good optician to a truly great optician in the mind of the patient. Remember from our previous discussion; Patients do not care how much you know until they know how much you care. Keeping them updated on their glasses is showing how much you care.

There is a constant battle between two forces after the patient makes the purchase. That of you proving yourself as a caring patient advocate versus the patient expectation that you are going to be just another average order taker. If a patient calls you to check on the status of their glasses, you have just lost the battle. You are no longer the caring optician. If, however, you can preempt this phone call by the patient with a call from you to the patient, the victory belongs to you!

The problem in most optical boutiques is that there is no system in place to make sure these phone calls get made. Typically, an optician will only call a patient when the glasses are ready to be picked up. If there is any communication with the patient about delayed orders it is up to the patient to call the optician. Well, you are not "most" opticians. You are a great one. Therefore, you do have a system in place to insure you call patients about their orders before the patient calls you. "I do have a system for this?" you ask. Yes, on a following page. Tear this out, make copies, and use it for every patient you see. Here's how:

In the first column, record the date the order is made. This will be the basis for all of your follow up calls. It is the day you and the patient sit down together and create their new pair of glasses. In the next column, the patients name to help you track the order followed by the date the order is placed. The "Order Placed" column is the day you send the information to the lab for fabrication. This helps you remember not to forget such an important task.

The columns for "Follow-up Call #1" and "Follow-up Call #2" are used to record when your preemptive call is made to the patient to either let them know the order is on track to be delivered as promised or has been delayed for some reason. The time separation between the "Order Date" and Follow-up Call #1 and between the two follow-up calls can be made to be anything you feel is appropriate for your office, however do not make these calls be more than 5 days apart. Anything more than five days and the patient's finger is going to start itching to call you. You need to make your preemptive call before this happens!

The "Dispense Date" column is for the day you give the finished glasses to the patient.

The "Satisfaction Call" is the nail securing you in the patient's mind as a *great* optician. This call is much underused in the industry and is likely the only time your patient has ever received such a call. It is a phone call made to the patient one week after they pick up their glasses to ask how they are adapting. This call is a win-win for everyone for several reasons.

1.) It gives the patient the impression that your optical boutique is not like any other they have been to. Even if they are happy with their glasses, it differentiates you from your competition.

2.) If they *are* having any difficulties, it allows you to invite them back to the office for a check of the glasses or adjustment before they revert back to their old glasses, complain to their neighbor, and go someplace else next year.

3) Most importantly, it allows you to remind the patient of the benefits gained by using your optical boutique. Emphasize the benefits of any premium options purchased, warranties, and ability to return to your boutique for free cleanings or adjustments as needed. This will keep the patient loyal to you even when being bombarded by ads from competitors. The patient will remember why they made the right choice to go to you.

My Patient Tracking Sheet

Optician _____

Order Date	Patient Name	Order Placed	Follow-Up Call #1	Follow-Up Call #2	Dispense Date	Satisfaction Call

Goal Setting Your Way to Greatness

Goal setting will be your single greatest work before all others in ascending from a good optician to a great one. A well designed goal is a paved road ahead of you guiding you to your destination. Earl Nightingale, the noted personal achievement coach, stated it well when he said "People with goals succeed because they know where they are going. It's as simple as that." It actually *is* as simple as that. You are going to end your day, your week, and your year somewhere. Wouldn't you want to be in control of where that somewhere is? Every road leads somewhere, this section is designed to help you pick the road that's right for you and see that you not only stay on course, but reach the end on schedule.

Do goals work? A recent study completed on Yale graduates answers this question. During school, only 3% of the study participants had kept a list of well defined goals for their school years and beyond. Twenty years later, the study was followed up with an assessment of their net worth. The 3% who had kept goals had a greater total net worth than the entire 97% of the graduates who had not. Granted, accumulating net worth is not the only way to measure success, however, this study does illustrate that for a given measure of performance, having a goal is invaluable.

Reading this book shows that at least you have some goal in mind to become a better optician. Is reading this book going to help you achieve that goal? Maybe, but only if you have the right motivation. Becoming the President, a doctor, an astronaut, a billionaire, or a great optician are all lofty goals, but they are not the right goal for everyone. In order for any goal to be achievable it must first be meaningful to you, not imposed upon you by someone else. This, however, does not imply that you can disregard the wishes of your managers. If it is meaningful to you for you to keep your job, and your boss gives you a deadline for a project, then that project deadline becomes a meaningful goal since you want to keep your job! The point here is whatever your goals may be, make sure you can verbalize the meaningful motivation behind them; otherwise it likely will not be achieved and will just waste your time in its pursuit.

Often, goal setting for someone is just having a vague idea in their head that, for example, "I want to be a better optician this year than last year". As we will learn, there is a science behind setting a good goal. We will discuss the four steps of creating a good goal and the four steps in making it happen. Don't worry if you don't memorize these steps, a *Goal Setting Worksheet* is provided at the end of this section to help you on your way to setting and achieving your goals, no matter how big or small.

The four parts of a goal

1. Make it Meaningful

If being a better optician is something you wish to attain (as reading this book would suggest) and you wish to set a goal to help you attain that, then the first question you must ask is why? Why do you want to attain this goal? The more personal the reason you have the more motivating the goal will be. There is no right answer, but make sure you know what "lights your fire" in your pursuit of the goal. Is it to make more money to support your family or take a long awaited vacation? Is it to be named Optician of the Year to make your family proud? If you have to think too hard about this there probably is not sufficient motivation behind your goal. Try a different goal.

2. Make it Specific

A goal of "wanting to be a better optician" or "make more money" isn't a specific enough goal to make it a reality. How do you define "better" Is it in selling more second pairs or in increasing your average dollar sales, therefore a reflection of getting to know your patients better? Is it reducing your avoidable remakes, such as incorrect PD measurements or matching the wrong prescription with frame style? If your goal is to make more money, how do you define more? How much more? $100 more than last year? 10% more than last year? How you define it does not matter, it will be different for everyone, just make sure you know the measure by which your goal will be evaluated and that it is appropriately linked with your meaningful motivation. For example, if your motivation for making more money this year is to buy your dream car, your specific goal had better make you enough money to be able to finance the payments!

3. Make it Measurable

For a goal to be attainable, you need to be able to measure its success. A goal of, for example, "increasing the number of referrals I get from previous patients by 10% this year" is a very specific goal, but is it measurable? It may be, but only if two conditions apply. 1) You know what you accomplished in this area last year and 2) you can continue to track referrals in the coming year. For such a goal, you would have to have had a good referral log from the previous year to know exactly how many patient referrals you had. Additionally, you would want to make sure to continue such a referral log into this year.

What if, using this goal, you do not have adequate referral records from the previous year to measure a 10% increase? It may be best then to revise your goal to read "I will increase my patient referral base by 10% each month this year using a patient referral log to track my referral sources." Such a goal is measurable even without any previous records because you are using the first month of your record keeping as the basis from which you grow 10% per month.

Goals often fall short of what they could achieve simply because the goal setter either does not make it measurable or sets the measurement bar too low. Remember to set your goal realistically, but do not short change yourself.

4. Make it Timely

Goals are not to be set for an indefinite period of time. There must be a time frame in which you hope to accomplish your goal. "Work will expand to fill the time allowed for its completion" is a quote that describes what will happen when working towards a goal with no deadline. Your goal needs to include a date on which you measure your success in achieving your goal.

Here are a few example of well written goals:

1) I will increase my 2nd pairs (specific) by 10% (measurable) for the year ending 2009 compared to 2008 (timely) so that I can qualify for the year end bonus and make a down payment on that new car.

2) I will have my bonus (specific) increase 7% (measurable) this quarter compared to this quarter last year (timely) so that I can take that trip to Las Vegas (motivation)

3) I will increase my average dollar sale (specific) 25% each month (measurable) going forward compared to last year (timely) so that I can justify to my boss allowing me to take Fridays off to spend time with my ailing mother (motivation).

While having an attainable goal with all above attributes does not by itself make it happen, it certainly helps. Now that we have a well conceived goal, how do we make it happen and turn this goal into a reality?

The four steps to make your goal a reality

1. Write it down

Simple yes. And absolutely necessary. A written goal is significantly more likely to be accomplished than one that is not written down.

2. Post it in a spot where you will see it daily

Tape it to the front of your computer screen. A refrigerator works well, too. Seeing it in print every day will rejuvenate, energize, and organize your thoughts around making the goal a reality. See, we are already through the first two steps and it has only taken you about 5 minutes.

3. Study what will be required

This is where the rubber meets the road. Prepare to meet your goal the same way you would prepare for a presentation, your retirement, or a job interview. Luck is never involved in achieving a goal. "Good luck" is commonly heard coming from acquaintances when you tell them of a goal. "Good Prepare" should be the mantra instead. This stage is the bulk of the work in meeting your goal. To take your performance to the next level in achieving your goal you will have to do something different than you have been. You cannot keep doing the same thing, using the same techniques, and expect a different outcome.

If your goal is to increase your second pairs by 10% over last year, you are going to have to learn some sales techniques (hopefully you already learned some from this book) which are different than the ones you are currently using. Ask your manager for help in sales techniques and use any number of available resources to help improve sales techniques. Don't think just within the optical world when looking for resources. There are many great books on helping you improve your general sales techniques no matter what field you are in. Just check your local bookstore. The bigger your goal, the more new techniques you are likely to have to learn. To increase your sales 5% you may need only one new technique, to increase it 20% you will need three or more new techniques.

A second aspect of this stage is in creating a flowsheet to help you identify the mini-steps needed to meet your goal. The bigger the goal, the more of these mini-steps there will be in your flowsheet. For example, if your goal is to become ABO certified, you will need to acquire study materials, apply for the test by the deadline, make time to study, and so forth. Making a list of these events will insure that you do not to miss a deadline and help to identify where bottlenecks may occur in your progress.

4. Measure progress

In order to achieve a goal, you must make an effort to measure your steps toward the goal. If a goal is set to be completed a year away, is can be hard to judge whether you are on track to complete it on time or not. Breaking it down into smaller monthly chunks so that you know if you are on track or need to speed up your work can be helpful.

On the next pages, you will find the *Goal Setting Worksheet*. Tear it our and make copies for each of your goals and enough for all your future goals. It is strongly recommended that you get yourself a goal setting book from your bookstore or library to learn more about the power of goal setting and other techniques to make them a reality.

Set goals for your professional life *and* personal life. Too often people wrap their identity around what they do for a living and fail to set goals for personal fulfillment. A person happy and fulfilled in their personal life will be a happy and fulfilled optician. Remember, despite the fact that it may feel like you spend most of your life at work, you are not your work. You are greater than your work. You need to cultivate relationships, achievements, and dreams outside work or risk never realizing your own personal greatness.

Goal Setting Worksheet

Writing your goal

1. What (SPECIFICALLY) do you want to accomplish?

_____

_____

_____

2. How am I going to measure success (MEASUREMENT)

_____

_____

_____

3. In what time frame will I complete this? (TIMELY)

_____

_____

4. Why do I want to accomplish this? (MOTIVATION)

_____

_____

_____

Preparing your goal

What steps need to be undertaken in order to reach your goal?

_____

_____

_____

_____

_____

_____

_____

Achieving your goal

Professional Goal: _____   **Deadline:**_____

Step 1: _____   Deadline:_____

Step 2: _____   Deadline:_____

Step 3: _____   Deadline:_____

Step 4: _____   Deadline:_____

Step 5: _____   Deadline:_____

Completion:_____

Personal Goal _____   **Deadline:**_____

       Step 1: _____   Deadline:_____

       Step 2: _____   Deadline:_____

       Step 3: _____   Deadline:_____

       Step 4: _____   Deadline:_____

       Step 5: _____   Deadline:_____

Completion:_____

Test Answers

Chapter 1 Answers

1. The cornea provides a clear window in the eye to allow images to pass through to the image processing tissue, the retina.
2. The optic nerve is the information superhighway of the eye. It transmits the information the retina collects and sends it to the brain for processing.
3. The image must be brought to a point of focus (the lens of the eye or a camera is responsible for this), and the image must be brought to focus on a surface capable of capturing the image in a form that either is saved (such as the film of a camera) or instantly processed (such as the retina of the eye).
4. The focal length is found using the equation $F = 1 / d$, where F is the power of the lens and d is the focal distance in meters. Therefore, $4 = 1 / d$. Solve for d and you have 0.25 meters or 25 centimeters.
5. Trifocals and progressives both have focal points for distance, intermediate, and near.
6. Lens
7. Astigmatism
8. Nearsighted (Myopia)
9. Plus power lens
10. -3.00 -1.00 × 180. 1) Add the sphere and cylinder together to get the new sphere. 2) Change the sign of the cylinder. 3) The axis is 90 degrees away from the original axis.
11. Five times worse. A 100-size letter is five times larger than a 20-size letter.
12. No. Only magnifiers magnify. Despite what you may hear, there are no such things as "magnifying glasses." Reading glasses, or "magnifying glasses," simply clarify reading material at a close distance, giving the illusion of a magnification effect.

Chapter 2 Answers

1. See your optical manager.

2. Step 1) Place glasses on patient's face. Step 2) Mark the location of the pupil with a Sharpie pen. Step 3) Place the lens in the lensometer and read the prism amount.

3. 3.6 prism diopters Base-in. Prism = F × D, so in the right eye Prism = 5 × .3 = 1.5, and in the left eye, Prism = 7 × .3 = 2.1. With a displacement of the optical centers outward in each eye and a minus-power lens, this places the thick part of the lens, the base, inward relative to the pupil in each eye. The horizontal prism is additive, so 1.5 BI plus 2.1 BI gives a total of 3.6 prism diopters BI.

4. Using a lens clock to measure the base curve in more than one axis of the lens. If the curves are different, warpage is present.

5. +1.50 to +2.00

6. The brand so that you can select the appropriate template for marking power locations.

7. Lens clock

8. Identifies the pupil location.

Chapter 3 Answers

1. Temple
2. Rounded edges, plastic to hide thick lens edge, small size
3. Rounded edges, rim all the way around the lens, small size
4. Weight of glasses
5. Safe and durable
6. Double bridge
7. A frame with a dark bridge
8. Frame PD

Chapter 4 Answers

1. Adjust the frame.
2. Pupillary Distance (PD)
3. Measuring PD
4. c. The proposed working distance.
5. The lower eyelid.
6. The center of the pupil.
7. The three-point touch.
8. Adjust the left temple inward or the right temple outward.

9. 10 degrees.
10. Spread the nosepads, increase pantoscopic tilt, and decrease vertex distance.
11. Well-made measurements

Chapter 5 Answers

1. Polycarbonate
2. Better vision without glare and better cosmetic appearance
3. Polycarbonate, as with most higher index lenses, have less light transmission and a higher Abbe value (more aberration). An antireflective coating will both increase light transmission and reduce aberrations in these lenses.
4. 1.66
5. Aspheric
6. The flat aspheric lens will increase reflections.
7. If the specific gravity is higher in the higher index lens.
8. Add an antireflective coating.
9. A flatter lens causing lash-crash and greater reflections.
10. Tint and UV coatings
11. Reduces reflections off the dark surface
12. Advantages: The spot on the lens is in focus for every distance in space, and there are no lines as there are in bifocals and trifocals.

    Disadvantages: Peripheral distortions and a smaller reading area than in conventional bifocals or trifocals.

Chapter 6 Answers

1. Advantages of hard lenses: Best optical quality, long lasting Disadvantages of hard lenses: Initial comfort, lacks disposability Advantages of soft lenses: Disposable, good initial comfort Disadvantages of soft lenses: Lack optical quality for irregular prescription
2. Removing a hard contact lens once you have visually verified that the lens is on the eye.
3. No. Cleaners remove debris, disinfectors kill germs.
4. Re-clean the lens at the end of every week. At the end of the month,

replace the case. Re-clean the lens again no more than forty-eight hours prior to lens wear.

5. Tyler's Quarterly

Chapter 7 Answers

1. "Film over eyes"; Dimness of colors; Blurry/Foggy vision; increased glare, especially at night.
2. Straight lines appear wavy; images disappear when focused upon; Blurry/Foggy vision.
3. Floaters
4. There are typically no symptoms in early-stage glaucoma.

Chapter 8 Answers

1. 2 diopters of prescription difference between the two eyes.
2. Slab-off. Contact lenses, separate reading and distance glasses, or a high-places bifocal segment are other less frequent alternatives to slab-off.
3. Equalize the center thickness the best as possible, equalize the base curve the best as possible, steer the patient to a small frame, and order slab-off if the patient is to wear a bifocal.
4. Slab-off is placed on the most minus, or least plus, power lens.
5. The blur from the cataract can hide the blind spot from macular degeneration. Once the cataract is removed, the macular degeneration blind spot may become more pronounced.

Chapter 9 Answers

1. Surfacing
2. Material, diameter, and base curve
3. Steeper
4. Generation
5. +3.00 D (+4.00 + (-1.00))
6. Fining and polishing
7. Edging
8. This is typically the antireflective coating not adhering to the lens. Although sometimes due to poor quality antireflective coating, many times it is from the lens still containing surface oils such as from fingerprints prior to the antireflective coating being applied.
9. Polycarbonate

About the Author

David S. McCleary, O.D., received his optomety degree from the Southern California College of Optometry. He currently is in practice with a large group, where part of his job involves training new and seasoned opticians hired into the practice.

Dr. McCleary has written and presented research at national meetings such as the American Academy of Optometry. In addition, the National Board of Examiners has selected him for the testing and licensure of new doctors.

He lives in Southern California with his wife, Laura, and daughter, Sarah.

For additional copies of this book, please visit www.opticiantraining.com

Index

Made in the USA
Las Vegas, NV
22 March 2023

69507427R00166